NEW PERSPECTIVES ON PUBLIC HEALTH POLICY

Issues in Policy History
General Editor: Donald T. Critchlow

NEW PERSPECTIVES
ON
PUBLIC HEALTH POLICY

Edited by
James Mohr

The Pennsylvania State University Press
University Park, Pennsylvania

This work was originally published as a special issue of *Journal of Policy History* (vol. 19, no. 1, 2007). This is its first separate paperback publication.

Library of Congress Cataloging-in-Publication Data.

New perspectives on public health policy / edited by James Mohr.
    p.   cm. — (Issues in policy history)

Includes bibliographical references.
Summary: "A collection of essays examining public health policy and the deci-sion-making process behind it"— Provided by publisher.
ISBN 978-0-271-02757-9 (pbk. : alk. paper)
1. Medical policy—History—20th century. I. Mohr, James C. II. Journal of policy history. III. Series: Issues in policy history (Unnumbered)
[DNLM: 1. Health Policy—history—Essays. 2. History, 20th Century—Essays. 3. History, 21st Century—Essays. 4. Policy Making—Essays.

WA 11.1 N532 2007]
RA393.N49 2007
362.1—dc22
2007043691

Series Editor Preface

Globalization in the twenty-first century has created new problems in public health. The free movement of goods and a migratory workforce allows for the quicker spread of pandemics and the introduction of new diseases to indigenous populations. Yet, while health problems have become globalized, health solutions remain local. As the authors of this volume observe, public health officials and health practitioners continue to operate within institutional and cultural settings unique to their countries and communities.

Furthermore, the globalization of health problems in the twenty-first century comes at a time in history when many of the older concepts of medicine, science, expertise, and public health have changed and indeed have eroded. The often-unquestioned faith that people had in progressive medicine and the advancement of science in the early twentieth century had diminished considerably by century's end. The erosion of this faith, as the authors in this volume explain, stems from multiple causes. The costs of public health are only one factor. Progressive medicine placed immense hope in the ability of medical and health experts to address complex problems in public health. While experts continue to play a vital role in medicine and public health, expertise in itself no longer carries the magic it once had. And much can be said similarly about science itself. The age of inevitable progress proved sanguine, even while science and medicine made revolutionary advancements.

The essays in this volume reveal the importance of the political, institutional, and general culture in which public health policies and programs are devised and implemented. Social and political conditions, institutional arrangements, racial and ethnic composition, and general values determine the conditions in which health policy develops and is implemented. As a consequence, public health needs to be studied within the context of culture. The essays in this volume impart an invaluable lesson for assessing previous public health policies and programs. Advances in public health will occur when public officials, health experts, medical practitioners, and the public understand the cultural environment in which public health operates in their nations, regions, and local communities. This volume argues for a tempered optimism concerning public health innovation and program development in the twenty-first century.

Donald T. Critchlow
Series General Editor

JAMES MOHR

Introduction: New Perspectives on Public Health Policy

The makers of public health policy face enormous challenges in the twenty-first century. In the past, their field has been imprecisely defined, deeply conflicted, poorly organized, and constantly changing. Lines of responsibility within the field are blurred at best, and groups with similar goals sometimes find themselves at cross-purposes. In the United States, state and local agencies interact with each other, with federal programs, and with powerful private interests. Many decisions that profoundly affect the health of the public are made for reasons largely unrelated to public health per se. Since the human and financial stakes involved in public health policies are immense, these challenges are, to say the least, serious issues. Underlying this volume is the belief that historical analyses and international perspectives can help policymakers understand, and hopefully begin to address, some of those old challenges in new ways.

The first two essays analyze what actually happened when two significant, well-intentioned public health initiatives were implemented on the ground in real-life situations. James Colgrove examines the tragic debacle that followed efforts to expand public health services in New York City during the 1960s, despite what appeared to be ideal conditions and an unprecedented infusion of federal funds. Virginia Berridge and Alex Mold explore similar developments in UK cities during the 1980s, when national health officials reoriented their approach to drug addiction. In neither case did the policies have the intended results, and these authors explain what actually happened and why. Both articles are cautionary tales that reemphasize the need for policymakers at the national level to understand the specific cultural and historical realities with which they are dealing.

The next three essays look at some of the factors that have determined how public health policy has actually been made in the past. Howard Kushner explores the role of powerful drug companies in the United States,

and raises the chilling prospect that their already self-interested activities in
the field of public health policy may have been operating historically within
a set of widely accepted assumptions that were fundamentally flawed in the
first place. Constance Nathanson examines the contingent nature of expertise in the formation of public health policy in the United States, the UK, and
France, showing the different ways in which policymakers in those nations
determined the "best" way to deal with two public health issues they all faced:
antismoking and AIDS-prevention programs. In the third essay, Harold
Pollack illustrates one of Nathanson's conclusions by showing how policies
designed to help intellectually disabled persons in the United States emerged
not primarily from governmental or professional initiatives, but in large part
from shifts in public perception and the pressure of grassroots organizations.
Although largely successful, that ad hoc process also had its own strengths
and weaknesses.

In the final essay, Brett Walker uses contemporary system theory to
illustrate six intriguing ways in which socioeconomic decisions in the past
have affected the long-term environmental health of Japan. By implication, of course, the makers of public health policy elsewhere need to
consider similar dynamics in their own nations as well. Together, these
six essays reveal important interactive factors that have influenced the
history of public health policy, and they help to situate the making of
public health policy in a transnational context.

University of Oregon

JAMES COLGROVE

Reform and Its Discontents:
Public Health in New York City
During the Great Society

The health-care system was one of the most visible and contentious battlegrounds on which the social conflicts of the 1960s unfolded. To an unprecedented extent, health status—especially the stark disadvantage in access and outcomes for racial and ethnic minorities and the poor—became an object of public and governmental concern during the Great Society era, as clinicians, community activists, politicians, and policymakers sought to create new models of medical care that were more equitable and efficient than those of the past. The social science theories that informed the ambitious programs of Lyndon Johnson's administration gave an imprimatur to the idea that illness was both cause and consequence of the "cycle of poverty."[1]

The ferment of this period raised fundamental questions about the place of public health in American society. For most of the twentieth century, the public health profession, concerned with prevention rather than cure and population-level analysis rather than patient care, was institutionally weak compared with organized medicine, and it struggled to advance a community-focused mission in a civic culture that privileged individualism, the free market, and limited government. In the latter half of the 1960s, grassroots mobilization, coupled with federal and state commitments to health care for the poor, opened a window of opportunity in which public health professionals could argue that their field, by virtue of its unique perspective and experience, had a special role to play in health reform. But the social and political conditions that created this opening also served as countervailing forces that limited what was possible in the new environment.

Nowhere was this landscape more unsettled than in New York City, which had a long tradition of innovative public health activities. In the mid-1960s, the city became, in the words of an economist who advised Mayor John Lindsay's administration, "one of the country's chief laboratories" for testing a "commitment to the use of the public authority to accomplish social change."[2] As part of an effort, now largely forgotten, to rationalize the city's massive and unwieldy health bureaucracy, the Department of Health was consolidated into an omnibus agency that linked it closely with the city's powerful medical and hospital establishment. Department employees sought to use new funding streams and a more open social climate to advance an expansive vision of public health, and forged new relationships with doctors and community members, the two constituencies that had historically bounded their mission. But their efforts at reform were caught between political and economic pressures from "above" and radical resistance from "below."

The social policy innovations of the War on Poverty and the Great Society have been the subject of extensive historical analysis.[3] But this literature has given little systematic attention to the health-care arena and virtually no consideration to the role of public health.[4] The debates over the appropriate sphere of public health provide a unique vantage from which to gain a fuller understanding of key transformations in American society in the 1960s: the shifting relationship between citizens and government; the expansion of legislative efforts to address the problems of the poor and disadvantaged; the development of a discourse of "rights," including the right to health; and the erosion of paternalistic notions of expertise, especially medical authority. This brief but pivotal chapter also sheds new light on challenges that still define the health-care system, as policymakers continue to debate the place of prevention within the country's technocratic and curatively oriented medical regime.

The Divergence of Public Health and Medicine

The professional and conceptual borders between public health and medicine were erected early in the twentieth century as clinicians in private or hospital practice diverged from sanitary reformers and laboratory-oriented bacteriologists in the public and voluntary sectors. As Allan Brandt and Martha Gardner have argued, the American health-care system was thus shaped by "the division of labor, the differences in theories and skills, and the balance of authority and politics between these two fundamentally related fields."[5] Physicians, represented by their increasingly powerful lobby, the American Medical Association, claimed authority over the domain of patient care and vehemently opposed moves by municipal and state health departments to provide clinical services.[6] As preventive practices such as routine physicals became common in the 1920s, public health officials clashed with doctors in private practice over who would deliver these services. These tensions crystallized in the debates over the publicly funded maternal and child health programs of the federal Sheppard-Towner Act, which Congress passed in 1921 and AMA lobbying killed eight years later.[7] In the decades that followed, public health became a kind of residual category: anything related to the population's physical well-being that remained outside the purview of organized medicine. Its practitioners collected statistics to map and control the spread of illness, published health-education materials, and performed a grab-bag of licensing and regulatory functions in areas such as restaurant sanitation. Their direct-care responsibilities were limited to poor charity patients who could not afford the services of a private physician, and treatment for tuberculosis and venereal diseases, stigmatized conditions for which they had historically been responsible.[8] The profession's heterogeneous workforce of doctors, nurses, epidemiologists, and educators claimed a more enlightened, sociologically informed view of health than the narrow focus of biomedicine, but their lack of political influence constrained their ability to shape the health-care environment.[9]

In the 1930s and 1940s, argues Elizabeth Fee, debates continued within the American Public Health Association "between 'progressives' who wanted public health and medical care services to be provided in a single, unified system and 'conservatives' who wanted to leave well enough alone: to confine public health to its traditional preventive activities and categorical programs, while leaving medical care to the clinicians."[10] In the postwar years, the growth in the biomedical research enterprise, exemplified by the dramatic rise in federal funding for the National Institutes of Health, reinforced the paradigm that illness was to be fought at the physiological rather than the societal level, and further eclipsed the perspective offered by the public health profession. The delivery of medical care remained firmly entrenched in a fee-for-service model, especially after the ignominious defeat of Harry Truman's proposal for national health insurance at the hands of the AMA. The association's strategy of hanging the label of "socialism" on any proposal for publicly funded health care successfully defused such initiatives through the 1950s.[11]

The emergence of poverty as a focus of the Kennedy administration set the stage for a reexamination of the status quo that had prevailed for decades. New legislative and policy initiatives addressed a set of related empirical and philosophical questions: How do poverty and its attendant social conditions influence health? How should medical care be linked not just with prevention but with housing, education, employment, and other aspects of welfare broadly conceived? What is the role of the state in providing some or all of these services? When Lyndon Johnson declared the War on Poverty in 1964, new health-related programs, premised on sociological and economic theories, poured money and expertise into communities around the country.[12] During Johnson's administration, Congress passed approximately fifty pieces of legislation related to health, providing funds that flowed through units of the federal government including the Office of Economic Opportunity (OEO), the Children's Bureau, and the U.S. Public Health Service. Annual federal spending on health grew from about $3 billion in 1959–60 to about $21 billion in 1970–71.[13]

The neighborhood health centers, funded by the OEO, were in many respects emblematic of the era. The centers were innovative demonstration projects designed to provide integrated medical screening, diagnosis, and treatment closely linked with ancillary services such as job training that would improve the life prospects of those attending. The centers' guiding principles included strong involvement of community members as advisors and lay workers; by explicitly seeking to foster the political empowerment of patients, they were intended to serve not merely as sites for care but as engines of social change.[14] In 1965 and 1966 the first round of eight centers opened, followed by another thirty in 1967 and 1968.[15]

The neighborhood health centers did not emerge from the federal public health establishment, though they embodied the philosophy of many of the field's liberals. Jack Geiger and Count Gibson, the Tufts University physicians who were architects of the neighborhood health center model, originally asked the Public Health Service to serve as a home for the program, but the agency, long reluctant to antagonize the medical lobby, referred the two men to the Office of Economic Opportunity.[16] It was unclear, moreover, whether the new federal interest and funding would strengthen the institutional position of public health, at least in its traditional bastion of state and local health departments. The OEO made most grants for neighborhood health centers to medical schools and hospitals, on the grounds that they were best positioned in terms of facilities, equipment, and clinical expertise to get up and running quickly. As a result, some public health officials saw the centers as undermining their status as the group best qualified to care for the poor.[17] In addition, the availabilityof health-related funding to nonprofit community-based organizations and other lay providers threatened to further splinter the field of public health, and dilute its already limited political influence, by adding to the diversity of the people addressing the connections among health, poverty, and social conditions.[18] Much was in flux in the new environment, and it was far from certain what role public health professionals would play in the reforms that seemed to be taking shape.

A Window of Opportunity and a Model for Reform in New York City

The New York City Department of Health seemed ideally positioned at the start of the Johnson administration to capitalize on the new policy environment. The department, a leader in the field since its founding as the country's first permanent municipal health authority in 1866, had established pioneering programs in health education, public health nursing, well-child care, and infectious disease control, and operated a network of twenty-seven health centers throughout the five boroughs that gave it a high profile in the community. But these centers reflected a long-standing accommodation with the city's private practitioners: they provided prevention and screening, but their clinical services were narrowly confined to the traditional categories of tuberculosis and venereal disease. Any other medical problem uncovered at a municipal health center was referred elsewhere—to a private doctor or hospital outpatient department—for follow-up and treatment.

When the neighborhood health center program emerged from the OEO, its principles resonated strongly with a cadre of health department employees dissatisfied with the sharp institutional boundaries between public health and medicine and the high concentration of preventable illness in the city's poor neighborhoods com+pared to its wealthy areas.[19] These employees were not radicals but career public servants for whom the new civil rights discourse of justice dovetailed with ideas about comprehensive care that they had formed after years on the front lines working with low-income populations. Theirs was a moderate, incremental vision of liberal reform, borne of the realism that came from working in the city's civil service. They sought mainly to broaden their traditional preventive activities to include ambulatory care, and secondarily to involve community members in the planning of services. But they did not see these changes as the gateway to radical social change or patients' political empowerment.

The department's most forceful advocate for expanding its provision of ambulatory care was Mary McLaughlin, an assistant commissioner. McLaughlin was a physician who had risen through the department ranks during two decades of service in poor neighborhoods. Her commitment and that of her like-minded colleagues grew in part from frustration at having to refer patients elsewhere for care, knowing that follow-through was unlikely because of costs and the fragmentation of the health-care system. In the fall of 1965 McLaughlin and her cohorts first requested funds from the City Council to expand the services of the district health centers beyond what they had traditionally offered to include a full range of outpatient care. The services would be provided by contracting with nearby hospitals, which would provide the clinicians and equipment. The first two sites chosen for the expansion would be in two of the city's most economically depressed neighborhoods, Bedford and Brownsville.

The budget request that the department submitted to the City Council reflected the ideals and language of the Great Society. It argued that "health and medical care programming must become very closely involved with social and welfare activities, public assistance programs and public housing, these in recognition that socio-economic factors are major determinants of health status."[20] The request also reflected the influence of the nascent consumer movement, which advanced the idea that health care was a commodity with which its purchasers had a right to be satisfied: "Health prevention and promotion on the one hand and diagnostic and curative services on the other," the document declared, "must be brought together into a more comprehensive non-fragmented, easily available package for the consuming public."[21]

Finally, in explaining its proposed partnership with hospitals to provide clinical services, the department contended that there was "an awakening and growing awareness by hospitals that their programs cannot remain parochial and unresponsive to the total health needs of their surrounding communities, and that they must be equal partners with the Health Department in the shaping of comprehensive health services for local communities."[22] There was little evidence of such an "awakening," and the assertion of one was rhetorical and strategic—designed to convince the City Council that the partnerships would bear fruit—rather than factual. The city's public and private hospitals (especially those in poor neighborhoods) had shown scant interest in the needs of their surrounding communities, and while they had cooperated in various health department initiatives, such as an ambulance transport service for premature newborns, they hardly viewed the health department as an "equal partner" in their work. To the extent that they were aware of the department at all, most hospital administrators viewed it as a civil service backwater far removed from the important business of patient care.

Even as this initial foray into ambulatory care was being made, the health department was facing an uncertain future. In 1965 the departure of George James, the popular commissioner, left a leadership void just as a major reconfiguration of the city's health bureaucracy was taking shape. As new debates unfolded about the professional spheres of public health and medicine, the existence of the department as a separate entity in city government was called into question. These developments in local politics were independent of the new federal health programs, but they would powerfully shape—and ultimately constrain—the incipient reform efforts that the department was undertaking.

John Lindsay and the Health Services Administration

On December 31, 1965, John Lindsay was sworn in as New York City's 103rd mayor. A charismatic liberal Republican and rising star on the national political scene, Lindsay promised to reform what he characterized as twelve years of corruption and complacency under Robert F. Wagner Jr. and the city's Democratic machine. He brought with him a team of "good government" planners armed with the latest ideas in municipal reform.[23] Health had not been a major issue during the campaign and was not high on the list of the new administration's initial priorities—relations with powerful labor unions took center stage when a strike by transit workers crippled the city on Lindsay's first day in office—but long-simmering problems, combined with new federal initiatives, soon pushed it to the top of the policy agenda.

When Lindsay took office, a profound sociodemographic shift was remaking the city, and the delivery of health services was becoming inseparable from issues of race, class, and poverty. Between 1950 and 1970 the city's white population declined by about 1.3 million, while its population of African Americans and Puerto Ricans increased by about the same number.[24] Many of these new arrivals were concentrated in slum neighborhoods, and their de facto primary-care providers were the understaffed and overcrowded emergency rooms and outpatient departments of the city's hospitals. Emergency-room visits to city hospitals doubled between 1960 and 1966.[25] Close to a third of the city's population, about 2.5 million people, were medically indigent.[26]

The magnitude of the city's health needs was matched by the size and complexity of its health-care sector, which accounted for about 15 percent of the city's $4 billion annual budget. Almost one in five of the city's 42,500 employees worked in either the department of health or the department of hospitals. The latter agency, established in 1929, ran nineteen hospitals and medical centers with some 18,500 beds. The city's department of welfare also ran seven clinics especially for welfare recipients.[27] Inefficiency, duplication of effort, and gaps in care were widespread. Both the health and the hospitals department operated bureaus of tuberculosis control, for example, which rarely communicated with each other. The department of welfare operated dental clinics for its clients only, while the health department ran dental clinics for children only, and the department of hospitals performed tooth extractions only.[28]

As part of their efforts to revitalize and streamline the city's civil service bureaucracy, Lindsay's team swiftly moved to consolidate some fifty municipal departments and agencies into ten "superagencies" that would unite related functions of government such as finance, housing, and transportation.[29] One of these was to be a new entity called the Health Services Administration (HSA), which would join the departments of health and hospitals under the same administrative umbrella. (The new organization would also include two other health-related agencies, the Community Mental Health Board and the Office of the Chief Medical Examiner. The Department of Welfare was made part of a different superagency, the Human Resources Administration.) While government reform was the chief impulse for the creation of the new agency, the proposed consolidation was consistent with one of the ideals that underlay the OEO's neighborhood health centers: that preventive and curative health services should be linked in a more continuous and patient-friendly system of care.

It was unclear, however, whether the organizational structure of the HSA would be a barrier or facilitator for the incipient movement within the health department to create new models of care. On the one hand, administratively uniting curative and preventive services seemed a logical and necessary step toward bringing about systemic change. The commissioners of all four of the affected agencies urged the City Council to pass enabling legislation, arguing that new federal grant programs made it essential for the components of the city's health-care system to become unified so that they would be well positioned to apply for funds that became available.[30] Mary McLaughlin, who championed the health department's involvement in clinical services, put the matter bluntly in a letter to the City Council: "The waste, duplication and inefficiencies of the past must come to an end."[31]

On the other hand, many public health leaders feared the dilution of what made their enterprise unique. Alonzo Yerby, a leading national figure in preventive medicine who had led the city's Department of Hospitals before taking a professorship at Harvard University, described this anxiety in an address at the Johns Hopkins School of Hygiene and Public Health in the fall of 1966: "Public health people fear that their preventive programs will be lost in the daily crises of providing hospital care for large numbers of patients. Administrators of public hospitals feel too hard-pressed by obsolete facilities, personnel shortages, strikes and work stoppages, and ever-mounting demands for services to consider the special needs of a program of prevention."[32] Said Cecil Sheps, a prominent hospital administrator and adviser to Lindsay, "When there's blood to stop flowing, and bones to mend, public health can get lost."[33]

Some of the uncertainty about whether the new HSA structure would impede or enhance reform involved the question of whether all organizational borders would be dissolved or whether the individual departments would be retained with a new layer of bureaucracy overlaid on top to coordinate their diverse functions. Members of the Board of Health, a five-member body made up of some of the city's medical and political elite, insisted in a letter to Lindsay that public health had to retain its independent status if the reform efforts were to succeed.[34] Lindsay promised the board members that reorganization legislation would specifically provide for a separate health department.[35]

Nevertheless, many health department employees remained anxious about their influence and their future. Their unease reflected in part the precarious position in which the department had only recently found itself. The department had enjoyed a heyday under the eight-year commissioner-ship of Leona Baumgartner (1954–62), who had assumed near-legendary status for her political savvy and tireless promotion of the department and its interests. When her widely respected successor, George James, resigned in 1965 to become dean of the Mt. Sinai School of Medicine, the department was suddenly without a strong leader to advance its interests as the merger took shape.

At the same time, pay stagnation created by a Lindsay administration salary freeze made it difficult to attract top-flight talent to the department's middle and upper ranks. The starting annual pay for an assistant commissioner in the Department of Health, a position that required a medical degree, was $25,000, compared to $27,500 for a master's level nonphysician administrator in the Department of Hospitals.[36] Many top managers left the health department following James's departure, while shortages of public health nurses—the department's "foot soldiers" against disease—left health centers understaffed and forced the cancellation of some programs, such as immunization clinics for low-income children. Working conditions in the district health centers, many of them deteriorating facilities that had not been renovated in decades, were difficult. "Years ago," wrote one health official, "the dynamic programming of the department with opportunity to do public health research as well as the desire of physicians to live in 'fun city' was sufficient to attract and keep staff. This is no longer true. Many now desire to leave the City where the problems sometimes seem insoluble and City living is no longer attractive."[37]

The extent of anxiety about the future was revealed by the unusual step taken by a group of health department physicians in the summer of 1966. Alarmed by the absence of a leader to serve as their advocate, they enlisted the assistance of former commissioner Leona Baumgartner, who remained an influential figure on the local health scene. "We feel that [creation of the Health Services Administration] will lead inevitably to a complete takeover of our department's functions by voluntary hospitals whose experience, goals and capabilities do not encompass the public health field at all," the doctors warned. "The end result of subordinating the Health Department's functions to those of hospitals will, we believe, result in a sharp curtailment or elimination of important preventive programs, a complete breakdown of department morale, and a resultant serious threat to the public health."[38]

The First Health Services Administrator

To fill the post of the city's first Health Services Administrator, who would be charged with fostering close relationships among departments that had operated with distinctly different missions and professional cultures, Lindsay's search committee turned to Howard J. Brown. An experienced program planner and manager as well as a physician, Brown had gained a strong reputation locally and nationally by designing an innovative outpatient clinic serving low-income residents of the city's Lower East Side that provided one of the models for the neighborhood health center program. He then went on to serve as the OEO's chief medical adviser, and helped establish similar facilities in rural Mississippi, in Watts, California, and in several other cities around the country.[39]

The choice of Brown thus provided a direct conceptual and practical link between New York City's health-care system and the reform initiatives emerging at the federal level. Brown's ideals were also consonant with those of the health department's progressives, who had taken steps to expand their ambulatory services, and his appointment augured well for these efforts. As Brown explained to Louis Craco, the young lawyer who chaired the Mayor's Task Force on Reorganization of the Government, shortly after accepting his new post: "There is a general consensus among modern public health and medical care professionals that the clinical, preventive and mental health services now fragmented should be united into coherent programs."[40] Preparing a statement that Lindsay would read in testimony before the U.S. Congress on health challenges facing the country's large urban areas, Brown identified the two most pressing problems as rebuilding deteriorating hospitals and financing and organizing medical care for "ghetto" areas.[41]

Not only was Brown committed to retaining an independent Department of Health within the HSA; he foresaw that it would be *primus inter pares* among the units that made up the combined organization. Describing his long-range vision of the mission of the department to colleagues at Johns Hopkins, Brown wrote, "The major planning, coordination, surveillance and evaluation responsibility of the total health programs in New York City" would rest with public health professionals, while the other units would have "more specialized functions, major as they will be, as compared to this broad charge of the Health Department."[42] The Department of Hospitals, he believed, would be limited to "bricks and mortar considerations." The health department's charge would not be "to do all that is necessary to protect and promote the city's health, but to make sure it is done" through standard-setting, surveillance, research, and demonstrations. Finally, he laid out a vision for the public health workforce that suggested a return to the social medicine roots of public health in the nineteenth century, when the field was guided by reformers such as Rudolph Virchow and Lemuel Shattuck. The public health leaders of the future, Brown predicted, would be "board certified public health physicians with training and skills in community medicine—medical sociologists, health urbanists—whatever they might be called . . . with one foot in the technical field of the science of medicine and the other in community dynamics."[43]

Brown's vision failed to thrive within the new bureaucracy, however. Almost immediately, differing institutional cultures and priorities and conflicting personalities resulted in turf battles involving authority over fiscal and programmatic matters among the four constituent agencies that had publicly supported the merger.[44] Brown found himself at odds with members of the medical establishment because of their unwillingness to embrace his view of health services organization. His increasingly blunt public criticisms of his fellow physicians—in one speech he contended that they organized care based on "their own need for professional distinction" rather than concern for patients—cost him critical support among what should have been a core constituency.[45] After seventeen turbulent months on the job, Brown abruptly resigned in December 1967.[46] Neither of his successors would last more than two years in the position. The lack of a consistent, forceful advocate at the helm of the Health Services Administration would prove to be a critical weakness that hampered the health department's ability to take the lead in reform.

"Ghetto Medicine": The Health Department as Care Provider and Watchdog

In spite of Brown's departure and the uncertain environment, health department employees committed to expanding the department's clinical services pressed ahead with their plans, fashioning a proposal for capital renovations of health centers that had previously provided only preventive services.[47] Because of the stigma that clung to free clinics for the poor, the new facilities would be named neighborhood family-care centers. "The term 'clinic' is scrupulously avoided in speaking of this program," Mary McLaughlin explained in a subsequent report. Each center would "operate on an appointment basis and we hope to pattern it on the type of care given in a private physician's office or a good group practice unit. The usual clinic appearance of benches, crowding, and lack of regard for patients' comfort, is a thing of the past."[48] After Lindsay's budget director and the City Council gave the go-ahead to the budget request to partially cover the substantial capital costs, plans for neighborhood family-care centers took shape. Seven would be in entirely new facilities and nine would be in renovations of existing sites in poverty areas.

That these forays by the health department into ambulatory care did not provoke the kind of resistance from the city's medical establishment that had been seen in the past is a testament to their incremental nature and the fact that they were limited to care for the poor, which was a traditional part of public health's purview. The lack of opposition also bespoke the degree of crisis in which the city's hospitals found themselves in the latter half of the 1960s. They had long been plagued by chronic staff shortages, deteriorating physical plants, and accusations of substandard care.[49] A mayoral task force appointed when Lindsay took office found rampant administrative inefficiency, wide disparities in the quality and quantity of preventive and curative services given to people of differing socioeconomic backgrounds, an unwillingness to adapt services to the needs of a racially and ethnically diverse patient population, and lack of outpatient-care facilities.[50] The modest effort by the health department to expand its ambulatory services in poor communities was, at that moment, the least of the hospitals' concerns.

Some resistance to the new neighborhood centers did come, however, from within the health department's own rank and file. The clinical staff of the health centers that were slated for expansion included many physicians with a more traditional orientation toward the appropriate spheres of public health and medicine. Because the new neighborhood family-care centers were to be operated in partnership with an affiliated hospital, many health department doctors feared that they would be subordinated in their work to better-trained hospital-based practitioners, or, worse, that they might be moved onto to the hospital payroll, thereby losing the seniority they had gained within the city's civil service system.[51]

A more serious threat to reform than resistance from within was the instability of funding. Reimbursements from Medicaid, the landmark federal-state program established in 1965 to finance care for the medically indigent, were expected to cover a major portion of the costs of the new clinical services.[52] But New York's Medicaid program had been in disarray virtually from its inception in 1966 due to unexpectedly high costs that had blindsided even knowledgeable insiders. Bureaucratic confusion reigned amid infighting over administrative matters such as patient eligibility and physician reimbursement.[53] In this precarious environment it was impossible to predict what level of funding would be available even a short time in the future; McLaughlin described the program's financing as "quicksand."[54] Indeed, in 1968 the parlous state of Medicaid set off a chain reaction that would reverberate throughout the state's health-care system, most powerfully in New York City. A pivotal point in the controversy was the state aid program known as "ghetto medicine."

The state department of health originated the ghetto medicine program in response to concerns about the shortage of medical care available to the poor in rural and urban slum areas. Two bills introduced in the New York legislature in the summer of 1968 amended the state public health law to allow local health departments to provide clinical services and to receive reimbursement from the state for fifty percent of their costs, the same proportion they received for their traditional categorical programs related to tuberculosis and venereal disease. The bills slipped under the radar of the large health-care interests and passed the legislature late in the session without debate.[55] McLaughlin submitted several applications for ghetto medicine funding to support the new neighborhood family-care centers, three of which were funded.

Within a year, however, the ghetto medicine program was unexpectedly transformed by the crisis of spiraling costs that had gripped New York's Medicaid program. By 1968, New York City accounted for fully one-quarter of the nation's total Medicaid enrollment and one-fifth of the total national expenditure on the program. Some 2.5 million residents—more than 30 percent of the city's population—had enrolled.[56] In response to the upwardly spiraling costs, the state legislature made drastic cutbacks in eligibility, resulting in close to 1.8 million adults and children being thrown off of the rolls. ("As a result of the confusion and despair regarding eligibility for medical benefits," cautioned a health department report in the summer of 1968, "we may one day very soon witness the first demonstrations for the right to health care in the United States.")[57] Although some of these individuals were subsequently re-enrolled, the overall rolls dropped by close to one million recipients, including almost three hundred thousand children.[58]

Faced with a fiscal crisis because of the sudden loss of revenue they had anticipated from Medicaid, many of New York City's private hospitals were forced to take out loans at high interest. The city's powerful hospital lobby enjoyed close access to Governor Nelson Rockefeller, and in the midst of the crisis sent representatives to meet with him to say they faced ruinous losses that could force the closure of some of their outpatient services.[59] State legislators agreed to use state aid through the ghetto medicine program to keep these hospitals' ambulatory-care services from going bankrupt. Thus money that had originally been intended to allow health departments to create new outpatient services for the poor was instead diverted to propping up existing services in private hospitals.

Liberal health advocacy and civic organizations were dismayed. They dubbed the plan "Operation Bailout" and claimed that private institutions with abysmal track records in caring for the poor should not be receiving public funds.[60] But faced with a more skilled and better-connected lobby, public health had been outflanked. A highly critical analysis by a member of the Citizens Committee for Children charged that public health "did not wish to take on the voluntary hospital establishment or else did not know how to do it. . . . Public health leadership was invisible, seemingly unable or unwilling to compete in the political arena."[61]

The diversion of money to the voluntary hospitals did come with strings, however, which McLaughlin and another assistant commissioner, Lowell Bellin, were successfully able to manipulate. In order for the hospitals to be eligible for state aid, they had to become "public" institutions. Their ambulatory-care services were therefore "municipalized" and placed under the aegis of the city heath department.[62] McLaughlin and Bellin quickly realized that the arrangement provided them with a wedge they could use to improve the services in institutions whose practices had long remained outside their managerial purview. As Bellin explained in a subsequent report, the ghetto medicine program allowed the department to use its "newly acquired fiscal leverage to accelerate socially desirable policies and administrative changes in voluntary hospitals historically insulated from health department dissatisfactions and restiveness."[63] Among the changes in policy and practice that the department included in the contracts they negotiated with each institution were the hiring of a director specifically responsible for outpatient care, the provision of interpreters for patients, development of lists of available services, and the convening of regular public hearings on matters of hospital policy.

Bellin's pursuit of oversight in private hospitals was consistent with a broader mission he had undertaken in 1967 to set standards and audit the quality of care provided by doctors participating in Medicaid. This watchdog role was made possible by a combination of legal and administrative authority: language in the Federal Title XIX (Medicaid) legislation, New York State's Medicaid law, and an administrative agreement between the city and state health department.[64] Bellin was aggressive and unapologetic in his vision of the health department's role in monitoring the provision of medical services. He drew an analogy to the department's other, well-accepted regulatory functions. "[The health department] furnishes a restaurant a license, which confers privileges," he explained. "It can always withdraw the license together with the privileges for due cause, that is, a cause in the interest of the public health. The analogy is obvious. The provision of foodstuffs to the public bears a potential hazard to the public health and therefore falls within the official purview of the local health department. Similarly, the provision of personal health services to the public bears potential hazard to the public health and therefore should fall within the official purview of the local health department."[65]

Unsurprisingly, Bellin experienced considerable pushback from local physicians. Typical was the complaint of the president of Queens Medical Society, who insisted that "quality medical care can no more be legislated than any Congress or Assembly or Senate can legislate honesty or integrity or tolerance."[66] A local medical society passed a resolution declaring itself "unalterably opposed to any system of self-imposed certification of a physician's competency by any governmental agency" and to "any governmental agency evaluating the quality of medical care."[67]

In spite of limited funding and personnel for enforcement, the health department's auditing and standard-setting program was one of its most successful reform efforts, sustained in large measure by the sheer force of Bellin's dogged personality. In 1969 rulings were handed down in three lawsuits challenging the department's authority to regulate tax-supported private medical care, and in each case the department's position was upheld. One concerned the reimbursement rate for chiropractic services; one challenged the authority to hold a hearing on allegedly fraudulent Medicaid dental services; a third affirmed the authority to suspend or eliminate podiatrists from Medicaid eligibility because of substandard care.[68]

The Perils of Community Involvement

As the health department confronted obstacles from "above"—lack of leadership in the Health Services Administration, the inadequacy of federal and state funding, and political maneuvering by the medical and hospital establishment—along with reluctance from within its own ranks, its reform efforts were simultaneously complicated by resistance from "below." Energized by the example of civil rights mobilization and challenges to long-standing power hierarchies, community groups contended, sometimes militantly, that they, not doctors, hospital managers, or health department bureaucrats, should have final say over how the city planned and delivered its health care. Although the department had actively sought to incorporate community input in the form of advisory boards for the new neighborhood family-care centers, the involvement of these groups added a new layer of dynamics with which the health department often found itself inadequately prepared to deal.

The input of "consumers" into the planning and implementation of services was a cornerstone of the Great Society's health programs. It was codified in federal legislation such as the Community Mental Health Centers Act of 1963, which mandated the creation of community advisory boards. This involvement was subsequently strengthened by the Office of Economic Opportunity's requirement for "maximum feasible participation" of poor communities in the neighborhood health centers.[69] In 1966, the Partnership for Health Act further institutionalized community-planning processes.[70]

Since the nineteenth century, New York City had had a well-developed voluntary sector of service organizations and civic groups concerned with health issues. Typical was the Citizens Committee for Children, which had been founded by a group of liberal social activists and philanthropists in 1946, and had a long track record of reform efforts, such as attempting to improve the conditions for African American youth in the city's notoriously segregated child welfare system.[71] In the 1960s, a new breed of community activist emerged. Unlike established organizations that grew out of a tradition of white protestant charity work by upper-class reformers, these new groups were more confrontational and less inclined to accomplish their goals by cultivating relationships with key decision-makers or engaging in time-consuming negotiation through official channels. Many groups were made up of the intended beneficiaries of services. As one observer summarized in 1969: "Frustration, confrontation, and overt conflict are more and more becoming the modes of problem-centered action by those interested enough to get involved. In the past, service projects were not cooperative ventures; they were imposed—albeit in a charitable way—from the one side, and the clients were at least expected to be happy with what they got. Today that is impossible. The new identity and increased self-esteem of the 'other America' has rejected the supplicant's role and demands more than charity."[72]

As the health department's neighborhood family-care centers took shape, citizens' groups subjected them to close scrutiny and, often, harsh criticism. In 1968, for example, the Citizens Committee for Children, the Lower East Side Neighborhood Association, and the Northeast Neighborhood Association wrote to Lindsay about "numerous complaints from community groups." The organizations claimed that the health department had failed to involve community members in the planning of services for centers that were being proposed for Harlem and Jamaica, Queens, and cited specifically the department's failure to clarify the standards for the services that would be offered in the new facilities and to provide ongoing information about their future plans.[73] The Citywide Health and Mental Health Council, another advocacy group, complained in a letter to Lindsay and the City Council that the Health Services Administration had displayed "a colossal disregard for community concern, dissent, and recommendation" and that the new organization had perpetuated "more of the same evils it was supposed to correct."[74]

The responsibility in the health department for day-to-day interactions with community groups typically fell to district health officers, physicians who earned relatively low salaries and were overburdened with other duties. Most were also white, older, and very different in socioeconomic background from the communities with whom they interacted. The complicated process of diplomacy and delicate negotiations, often racially charged, required a skill set very different from what they had developed in their professional training and experience.[75]

Pressure from liberal advocacy groups, including HealthPAC and the Citizens' Committee for Children, had led to a provision in the ghetto medicine legislation requiring that, in return for receiving state aid, each beneficiary hospital create an advisory board made up of fifty-one percent of its members from the community.[76] But the degree of authority these bodies would have over hospitals' decision-making, and indeed the precise nature of their mission, was ambiguous. According to the official guidelines promulgated by the city, the groups "should neither be interpreted as having 'community control' nor as performing a perfunctory role. The committee should be viewed as a mechanism to facilitate both delivery and community utilization of ambulatory services."[77] The health department was to work closely with the advisory groups, serving as a kind of mediator between their interests and perspectives and those of the hospitals. But these alliances were not uncomplicated. The committees varied widely in their knowledge of the health-care sector and their skill at dealing with the byzantine operations of hospitals. Mutual mistrust and even hostility characterized the relationships between some of the committees and the hospitals they advised; one committee filed suit against both the hospital and the health commissioner, claiming that they deliberately withheld needed information.[78]

Even as the health department's new involvement with medical care brought it into conflict with community groups, it also met resistance in its traditional domain of population-level prevention. Amid increasingly assertive grassroots activism, the department's efforts to address illnesses related to poor living conditions encountered a minefield of potential criticism. The challenges of dealing with a health problem that was both deeply entrenched in poverty and subject of militant community action crystallized around the issue of lead poisoning. In 1967, the city recorded 642 cases of lead poisoning—mostly among African American and Puerto Rican children—and four deaths.[79] Political pressure on the Lindsay administration to address the issue began to mount as an increasing number of citizens' groups began accusing the city of "genocide" of its poor children living in slum housing.[80] In response, the department undertook a pilot program evaluating the use of an experimental urine test that could be used in door-to-door screening to determine the extent of the problem and identify children in need of treatment. In 1969, a group of young student radicals and Puerto Rican nationalists, the Young Lords, mounted a public challenge to this effort.[81]

The Young Lords, in the tradition of militant activist groups such as the Black Panthers, sought to fight economic and political injustice and bring about radical social change. A New York chapter of the group, formed in 1969 after splintering from the founding organization in Chicago, first made a mark by collecting garbage from the sidewalks of East Harlem and piling it in the middle of the streets, forcing the department of sanitation to remove it so that traffic could flow. The garbage dumpings escalated over the summer of 1969 into demonstrations in which the Lords barricaded neighborhood streets and clashed with police. Soon after their formation, the group adopted the health of the residents of *el barrio* as a primary focus of their activism.[82] In the fall the group issued a "10-point health program" that included demands for "total self-determination of all health services in East Harlem" and "free publicly supported health care for treatment and prevention." The plan clearly revealed the extent to which poor health was viewed as inseparable from other forms of social injustice: one of the ten points demanded "education programs for all the people to expose health problems—sanitation, rats, poor housing, malnutrition, police brutality, pollution, and other forms of oppression." The plan also took direct aim at the city's existing health-care bureaucracy: point 2 demanded "immediate replacement of all Lindsay and [Hospitals commissioner Joseph] Terenzio administrators by community and staff-appointed people whose practice has demonstrated their commitment to serve our poor community."[83]

On the morning of November 24, 1969, about thirty people, mostly members of Young Lords and their supporters, arrived at health department headquarters. They entered the office of Mary McLaughlin—whom Lindsay had recently appointed health commissioner—demanding a meeting about the issue of lead paint. McLaughlin and the assistant commissioner in charge of lead poisoning were at an all-day conference across town, but the group insisted they would not leave the premises until their demands were met. They wanted the department to turn over some forty thousand urine test kits that were being used in the pilot screening program; convinced that the failure to deploy the kits more widely was rooted in indifference to the problems of poor ethnic minorities, the group sought to take matters into their own hands and do the outreach themselves. McLaughlin's secretary was able to reach one of her deputies, David Harris, who rushed to McLaughlin's office to meet with the group. With the demonstrators sitting on the floor or perched on tabletops, Harris explained that the test kits were of uncertain validity and were still being evaluated. A deal was ultimately reached to allow the Young Lords to use a limited number of kits in collaboration with health department doctors who had expertise in lead screening.[84]

The confrontation in the commissioner's office epitomized the clashing perspectives of health professionals and activists. Where Harris saw the need to proceed carefully according to scientific evidence so as not to waste scarce resources on measures that might be ineffective or counterproductive, aggrieved community members saw bureaucratic stonewalling. (The urine test, it was later confirmed, was not a valid predictor of lead poisoning and was thus unsuitable for use in a screening program.)[85]

In the aftermath of the occupation, the liberal weekly newspaper the *Village Voice*, which had given supportive coverage to the Young Lords' previous efforts, took up the cause of lead poisoning among ghetto children. Muckraking *Voice* columnist Jack Newfield, a crusader for liberal political causes, repeatedly pilloried Lindsay and the health department for their inaction. He charged that mayoral aid Werner Kamarsky and McLaughlin were "cut off from the dailiness of injustice by their positions and life styles"[86] and bluntly accused McLaughlin of lying to the mayor and the press about the extent of the lead paint problem and the department's response.[87]

The following summer, the city was rocked by repeated unrest in the city's poor African American and Puerto Rican neighborhoods. In June, angry residents of Brownsville burned garbage in the streets in protest of poor municipal services.[88] The same week, after one of the Young Lords' leaders was arrested, hundreds of youths rioted in East Harlem, smashing store windows and burning garbage. Three days after the riot, the Young Lords mounted another assault on health department judgment around another issue that disproportionately affected the poor: tuberculosis. On June 17, a group of Young Lords "liberated" a mobile tuberculosis screeing van parked at 116th Street and Lexington Avenue in East Harlem. After driving the van five blocks south and one block west, they parked it across the street from the group's headquarters, draped a Puerto Rican flag over it, and rechristened it the Ramón Emeterio Betances Health Truck, in honor of the nineteenth-century Puerto Rican doctor and antislavery revolutionary. The X-ray technicians inside continued to perform their duties as crowds milled around outside, television crews parked at the scene, and a heavy police presence gathered, including officers stationed on the roofs of adjoining buildings.[89] After several hours of tense negotiations involving the Lords, the health officer in charge of East Harlem, and department officials downtown, an agreement was reached stipulating that the truck would be free to travel "anywhere in the metropolitan area as deemed necessary by the Young Lords party for the best health care for our poor and oppressed people."[90]

Epilogue: The Limits of Reform

During the Great Society era, moderate liberals within the New York City health department were able to advance a variety of reforms within the progressive political and social climate that prevailed nationally. They added ambulatory care to their traditional preventive activities, involved community members in the planning and implementation of services, audited the quality of care provided by physicians receiving reimbursement from public funds, and mounted new efforts to address health problems such as lead poisoning that were rooted in socioeconomic injustice. At the same time, however, forces "below" and "above" constrained what they could accomplish. Community members newly empowered as partners in health department efforts often proved uncooperative and even hostile, while financing from federal and state legislation remained unstable. The crisis of New York State's unforeseen and exorbitant Medicaid expenses, it was clear in retrospect, doomed the funding for the health department's efforts. The subsequent diversion of state money from the department to private hospitals "took the heart out of the 'Ghetto Medicine' program," a subsequent analysis argued, "before it could be started."[91] Just three neighborhood family-care centers were created, far short of the sixteen originally envisioned.

Even more severe fiscal retrenchment would soon put a decisive end to reform. The continued flight of the middle class to the suburbs during the early 1970s and the consequent erosion of the tax base plunged New York City into straits that culminated in its infamous collapse into insolvency in 1975. The city was taken over mid-year by a "municipal assistance corporation" (dubbed "Big Mac" by local pundits), an independent coalition of investors that kept the city solvent by assuming the most immediate of its massive debts.[92] The staff of the Department of Health was cut by one-fourth. In a series of triage decisions, department services were categorized as "life saving" versus "life enhancing," with the latter subject to cuts.[93] In this environment, the kind of expansion that had become possible in the mid-1960s was foreclosed.

At national level, backlash against the "big government" solutions of the Johnson administration had begun to set in before they had scarcely gotten under way. Typical was the fate of the neighborhood health center program. Funding for the centers remained flat during the Nixon and Ford administrations, in spite of escalating health-care costs; beginning in 1970, the program was gradually transferred from the OEO to the Department of Health, Education, and Welfare, where it "stagnated," according to an analysis in the late 1970s.[94] As consequential as the lack of financial commitment was the disappearance of the political will to expand health and welfare services for the poor.

Even in New York City, with its tradition of liberalism and generous social provision, the public health profession's advocates for reform were hobbled by their institutional position: most were either political appointees or civil servants subject to pressure from powerful interests and lacking a natural base of constituents to support their work. As a result, their vision of change was realistic and incremental rather than radical. To some of the field's liberal members, this realism, placed against the promise of the Great Society's ambitious ideals, simply provided a cover for political timidity and ineptitude. This view was given voice most eloquently by Paul Cornely, a Howard University professor of preventive medicine. Newly elected in 1969 as the first African American to head the American Public Health Association, he gave an address at the group's annual meeting in Philadelphia in which he sharply chided his colleagues for their failure to advocate more aggressively for reform. Cornely declared that the association had been "a mere bystander" on urgent social issues such as occupational health and environmental protection, and had failed to put forth any concrete proposal for a national health plan during the preceding decade when the possibility of so much change had been on the table. Public health professionals, he charged bluntly, remained "outside the power structure."[95] But as the experience of New York City reveals, the prospects for public health professionals to grasp the levers of power were always limited, even at one of the most progressive moments of the twentieth century.

Mailman School of Public Health
Columbia University

Notes

1. Robert M. Hollister, Bernard M. Kramer, and Seymour S. Bellin, "Neighborhood Health Centers as a Social Movement," in Robert M. Hollister, Bernard M. Kramer, and Seymour S. Bellin, eds., *Neighborhood Health Centers* (Lexington, Mass., 1974). On the influence of social science research on Great Society programs, see Carl M. Brauer, "Kennedy, Johnson, and the War on Poverty," *Journal of American History* 69 (1982): 98–119.

2. Nora Piore, "Rationalizing the Mix of Public and Private Expenditures in Health," *Milbank Memorial Fund Quarterly* 46 (1968): 161–70; 168.

3. See, for example, Allan J. Matusow, *The Unraveling of America: A History of Liberalism in the 1960s* (New York, 1984); Ira Katznelson, "Was the Great Society a Lost Opportunity?" in Steve Fraser and Gary Gerstle, eds., *The Rise and Fall of the New Deal Order, 1930–1980* (Princeton, 1989); John Morton Blum, *Years of Discord: American Politics and Society, 1961–1974* (New York, 1991); Gareth Davies, *From Opportunity to Entitlement: The Transformation and Decline of Great Society Liberalism* (Lawrence, Kan., 1998); Maurice

Isserman and Michael Kazin, *America Divided: The Civil War of the 1960s* (New York, 1999); and Brauer, "Kennedy, Johnson, and the War on Poverty."

4. An excellent examination of liberal activists within the medical profession during this period is Naomi Rogers, "'Caution: The AMA May Be Dangerous to Your Health': The Student Health Organizations (SHO) and American Medicine, 1965-1970," *Radical History Review* 2001(80): 5-34.

5. Allan M. Brandt and Martha Gardner, "Antagonism and Accommodation: Interpreting the Relationship Between Public Health and Medicine in the United States During the 20th Century," *American Journal of Public Health* 90 (2000): 707-15.

6. John Duffy, "The American Medical Profession and Public Health: From Support to Ambivalence," *Bulletin of the History of Medicine* 53 (1979): 1-15; and Paul Starr, *The Social Transformation of American Medicine* (New York, 1982), 180-97.

7. Richard A. Meckel, *Save the Babies: American Public Health Reform and the Prevention of Infant Mortality, 1850-1929* (Baltimore, 1990); J. Stanley Lemons, "The Sheppard-Towner Act: Progressivism in the 1920s," *Journal of American History* 55 (1969): 776-86.

8. Paul Starr, *The Social Transformation of American Medicine* (New York, 1982), 180-97.

9. Daniel M. Fox, "The Politics of Public Health in New York City: Contrasting Styles Since 1920," in David Rosner, ed., *Hives of Sickness: Public Health and Epidemics in New York City* (New Brunswick, N.J., 1995).

10. Elizabeth Fee, *Disease and Discovery: A History of the Johns Hopkins School of Hygiene and Public Health, 1916-1939* (Baltimore, 1988), 231.

11. Starr, *The Social Transformation of American Medicine,* 280-86.

12. Byron G. Lander, "Group Theory and Individuals: The Origin of Poverty as a Political Issue in 1964," *Western Political Quarterly* 24 (1971): 514-26; Brauer, "Kennedy, Johnson, and the War on Poverty."

13. Robert Stevens and Rosemary Stevens, *Welfare Medicine in America: A Case Study of Medicaid* (New York, 1974), 45.

14. Karen Davis and Cathy Schoen, *Health and the War on Poverty: A Ten-Year Appraisal* (Washington, D.C., 1978), 161-73.

15. Hollister, Kramer, and Bellin, "Neighborhood Health Centers as a Social Movement."

16. Sar Levitan, "Healing the Poor in Their Own Back Yards," in *Neighborhood Health Centers.*

17. Alice Sardell, *The U.S. Experiment in Social Medicine: The Community Health Center Program, 1965-1986* (Pittsburgh, 1988), 60, 64-66.

18. Fox, "The Politics of Public Health in New York City."

19. Anthony C. Mustalish, Gary Eidsvold, and Lloyd F. Novick, "Decentralization in the New York City Department of Health: Reorganization of a Public Health Agency," *American Journal of Public Health* 66 (1976): 1149-54.

20. "Statement of the Department of Health on Its Proposed 1966-67 Capital Budget Request," typescript, 22 October 1965, New York City Department of Health Archives (hereafter NYCDOH), Box 141979, Folder: Budget–Capital.

21. Ibid. On the rise of the idea that patients were "consumers" of health care, see Nancy Tomes, "Patients or Health-Care Consumers? Why the History of Contested Terms Matters," in Rosemary A. Stevens, Charles E. Rosenberg, and Lawton R. Burns, eds., *History and Health Policy in the United States: Putting the Past Back In* (New Brunswick, 2006). On the consumer movement more generally in the years following World War II, see Lizabeth Cohen, *A Consumer's Republic: The Politics of Mass Consumption in Post-War America* (New York, 2004).

22. "Statement of the Department of Health on Its Proposed 1966-67 Capital Budget Request," 2.

23. Vincent Cannato, *The Ungovernable City: John Lindsay and His Struggle to Save New York* (New York, 2001).

24. Eli Ginzberg, *Urban Health Services: The Case of New York* (New York, 1971).

25. Commission on the Delivery of Personal Health Services, *Comprehensive Community Health Services for New York City* (New York, 1968).

26. Nora Piore to Joan Leiman, 25 October 1966, NYCDOH, Box 142000, Folder Budget General.

27. "Report of the Mayor's Advisory Task Force on Medical Economics," typescript, 14 February 1966, NYCDOH, Box 141998, Folder: Mayor.

28. Howard Brown to Louis Craco, 7 June 1966, NYCDOH, Box 142007, Folder: Mayor; HSA annual report for 1966.

29. Cannato, *The Ungovernable City*, 108–18.

30. Statement of Howard J. Brown to the Council of the City of New York, 13 September 1967, NYCDOH, Box 142017, Folder: HSA Reorganization.

31. Mary McLaughlin to Edward Sadowsky, 12 September 1967, NYCDOH, Box 142017, Folder; HSA Reorganization.

32. Alonzo S. Yerby, "Health Departments, Hospitals and Health Services," *Medical Care* 5 (1967): 70–74; 72.

33. Martin Tolchin, "Merger Put Off for 2 City Units," *New York Times*, 18 March 1966, 41.

34. Lewis Loeb to John Lindsay, 8 August 1967, NYCDOH, Box 142017, Folder: HSA Reorganization.

35. John Lindsay to Lewis Loeb, 21 August 1967, NYCDOH, Box 142017, Folder: HSA Reorganization.

36. Bernard Bucove to Edward O'Rourke, 15 February 1968, NYCDOH, Box 142238, Folder: Health Services Administration.

37. Ibid. The *New York Herald-Tribune* columnist Dick Schaap dubbed New York "fun city" soon after Lindsay was elected. Cannato, *The Ungovernable City*, 108.

38. Donald C. Meyer to Leona Baumgartner, 8 August 1966, NYCDOH, Box 142008, Folder: Baumgartner. See also Martin Tolchin, "City Health Aides Fear for Agency," *New York Times*, 25 October 1966, 33.

39. Ginzberg, *Urban Health Services: The Case of New York*; Howard J. Brown, *Familiar Faces, Hidden Lives: The Story of Homosexual Men in America Today* (New York, 1976).

40. Howard Brown to Louis Craco, 7 June 1966, NYCDOH, Box 142007, Folder: Mayor.

41. Howard J. Brown to Murray Drabkin, 10 August 1966, NYCDOH, Box 142002, Folder: Mayor.

42. Howard J. Brown to Sol Levine, 20 November 1967, NYCDOH, Box 142273, Folder: 10-Year Plan.

43. Ibid.

44. See, for example, the correspondence among Mayor Lindsay, Health Services Administrator Howard Brown, and Marvin Perkins, health of the Community Mental Health Board, August 1966, NYCDOH, Box 142000, Folder: Mental Health Board.

45. Martin Tolchin, "Dr. Brown Quits Post as City Health Chief," *New York Times*, 6 December 1967, 1.

46. Ironically, Brown's departure was unrelated to his management of the HSA. He was told by his brother-in-law, a *New York Times* reporter, that the investigative journalist Drew Pearson was planning to expose homosexuals in the Lindsay administration. Brown, a gay man whom the *Times* had coyly identified as a forty-two-year-old bachelor who lived in a Greenwich Village townhouse when it had announced his appointment, believed the public destruction of his reputation would cost him his ability to function effectively in the job. Six years later, Brown publicly came out and called on the City Council to pass antidiscrimination legislation covering sexual orientation. Brown, *Familiar Faces, Hidden Lives*, 15–18.

47. "HSA Annual report for 1966," typescript, NYCDOH, Box 142008, Folder: Health Department.

48. Mary C. McLaughlin, "Issues and Problems Associated with the Initiation of the Large-Scale Ambulatory Care Program in New York City," *American Journal of Public Health* 58 (1968): 1181–87; 1182.

49. Willard C. Rappleye, "The Hospitals of New York City," *Bulletin of the New York Academy of Medicine* 37 (1961): 525–30; Howard J. Brown, "Municipal Hospitals," *Bulletin of the New York Academy of Medicine* 43 (1967): 450–55.

50. "Report of the Mayor's Advisory Task Force on Medical Economics," typescript, 14 February 1966, NYCDOH, Box 141998, Folder: Mayor.

51. Ibid.

52. Ginzberg, *Urban Health Services: The Case of New York*, 155.

53. Stevens and Stevens, *Welfare Medicine in America*, 92–95, 109–12.

54. Mary C. McLaughlin, "Present Status and Problems of New York City's Comprehensive Neighborhood Family Care Health Centers," *Bulletin of the New York Academy of Medicine* 44 (1968): 1390–95.

55. Steven Jonas, "Organized Ambulatory Services and the Enforcement of Health Care Quality Standards in New York State," in Marvin Lieberman, ed., *The Impact of National Health Insurance on New York* (New York, 1977); Mary C. McLaughlin, Florence Kavaler, and James Stiles, "Ghetto Medicine Program in New York City," *New York State Journal of Medicine* 71 (1971): 2321–25; 2323.

56. Edward O'Rourke, "Medicaid in New York: Utopianism and Bare Knuckles in Public Health," *American Journal of Public Health* 59 (1969): 814–15.

57. "Position paper; Medicaid Program; New York City," typescript, 21 August 1968, NYCDOH, Box 142239, Folder: Medicaid.

58. Ibid.

59. Betty J. Bernstein, "What Happened to 'Ghetto Medicine' in New York State?" *American Journal of Public Health* 61 (1971): 1287–93; R. Andrew Parker, "The Case of Ghetto Medicine," in Herbert Hyman, ed., *The Politics of Health Care: Nine Case Studies of Innovative Planning in New York City* (New York, 1973).

60. Parker, "The Case of Ghetto Medicine."

61. Bernstein, "What Happened to 'Ghetto Medicine' in New York State?"

62. Mary C. McLaughlin, "Transmutation into Protector of Consumer Health Services," *American Journal of Public Health* 61 (1971): 1996–2004.

63. Lowell Eliezer Bellin, Florence Kavaler, and Al Schwarz, "Phase One of Consumer Participation in Policies of 22 Voluntary Hospitals in New York City," *American Journal of Public Health* 62 (1972): 1370–78.

64. Senate Committee on Finance, *Medicare and Medicaid: Problems, Issues, and Alternatives* (Washington, D.C., 1970), 249.

65. Lowell Eliezer Bellin, "Local Health Departments: A Prescription Against Obsolescence," *Proceedings of the Academy of Political Science* 32 (1977): 42–52; 49–50.

66. Murray Elkins to James Haughton, 28 April 1967, NYCDOH, Box 142014, Folder.

67. Martin Cherkasky, "Voluntary Hospitals," *Bulletin of the New York Academy of Medicine* 43 (1967): 456–62.

68. Lowell Eliezer Bellin and Florence Kavaler, "Policing Publicly Funded Health Care for Poor Quality, Overutilization, and Fraud—The New York City Medicaid Experience," *American Journal of Public Health* 60 (1970): 811–20.

69. Paul C. Nutt, "The Merits of Using Experts or Consumers as Members of Planning Groups: A Field Experiment in Health Planning," *Academy of Management Journal* 19 (1976): 378–94. The merits and drawbacks of community involvement have been subject to considerable analysis and commentary, perhaps most famously by Daniel Patrick Moynihan in his memoir of disillusionment, *Maximum Feasible Misunderstanding: Community Action in the War on Poverty* (New York, 1970).

70. Basil J. F. Mott, "The New Health Planning System," *Proceeds of the American Academy of Political Science* 32 (1977): 238–54.

71. Gerald Markowitz and David Rosner, *Children, Race, and Power: Kenneth and Mamie Clark's Northside Center* (Charlottesville, Va., 1996), 56–58.

72. Jeoffrey B. Gordon, "The Politics of Community Medicine Projects: A Conflict Analysis," *Medical Care* 8 (1969): 419–28; 422.

73. Citizens' Committee for Children, Lower East Side Neighborhood Association, and North East Neighborhood Association to John Lindsay, 6 February 1968, NYCDOH, Box 142240, Folder: Ambulatory Care.

74. A. Ruben Mora to Mayor, Members of the City Council, and Board of Estimate, 21 August 1968, NYCDOH, Box 142030, Folder: Legislation.

75. Mary McLaughlin to Edward O'Rourke, 14 February 1968, NYCDOH, Box 142240, Folder: Ambulatory Care.

76. Herbert Hyman, "The Unfulfilled Health Hopes in New York City," in Hyman, ed., *The Politics of Health Care*; Jonas, "Organized Ambulatory Services and the Enforcement of Health Care Quality Standards in New York State."

77. McLaughlin, Kavaler, and Stiles, "Ghetto Medicine Program in New York City," 2321–25; 2323.

78. Ibid.

79. Edward O'Rourke to Werner Kamarsky, 8 November 1968, NYCDOH, Box 142240, Folder: Environmental Health Services.

80. Ibid.

81. The group's origins are recounted in its own history: Young Lords Party, *Palante!* (New York, 1971). See also Jennifer A. Nelson, "'Abortions Under Community Control': Feminism, Nationalism, and the Politics of Reproduction Among New York City's Young Lords," *Journal of Women's History* 13 (2001): 157–80.

82. Young Lords Party, *Palante!*

83. "10-Point Health Program," flyer, NYCDOH, Box 142260, Folder: Bureau of Chronic Disease.

84. David Harris to Thomas Morgan, 10 December 1969, NYCDOH, Box 142276, Folder: Dr. Harris.

85. M. Specter, Vincent Guinee, and B. Davidow, "The Unsuitability of Random Urinary Delta Aminolevulinic Acid Samples as a Screening Test for Lead Poisoning," *Journal of Pediatrics* 79 (1971): 799–804.

86. Jack Newfield, "Fighting an Epidemic of the Environment," *Village Voice*, 18 December 1969, 12.

87. Jack Newfield, "My Back Pages," *Village Voice*, 25 December 1969, 24.

88. See, for example, Joseph Lelyveld, "Brownsville Erupts in Violence Over Huge Accumulations of Garbage," *New York Times*, 13 June 1970, 1; "Garbage Burned in East Harlem," *New York Times*, 4 August 1970, 18; "Community Groups Criticize Garbage Collections as 'Sporadic,'" *New York Times*, 6 August 1970, 25.

89. Thomas W. Jones to J. Warren Toff, 19 June 1970, NYCDOH, Box 142271, Folder: Tuberculosis; Alfonso Narvaez, "The Young Lords Seize X-Ray Unit," *New York Times*, 18 June 1970, 17.

90. "Agreement Between the Young Lords Party and the City Department of Health," 17 June 1970, NYCDOH, Box 142271, Folder: Tuberculosis.

91. Jonas, "Organized Ambulatory Services and the Enforcement of Health Care Quality Standards in New York State."

92. Steven R. Weisman, "How New York Became a Fiscal Junkie," *New York Times*, 17 August 1971.

93. Pascal James Imperato, "The Effect of New York City's Fiscal Crisis on the Department of Health," *Bulletin of the New York Academy of Medicine* 54 (1978): 276–89.

94. Davis and Schoen, *Health and the War on Poverty*, 170.

95. Paul B. Cornely, "The Hidden Enemies of Health and the American Public Health Association," *American Journal of Public Health* 61 (1971): 7–18.

ALEX MOLD and VIRGINIA BERRIDGE

Crisis and Opportunity in Drug Policy: Changing the Direction of British Drug Services in the 1980s

During the 1980s illegal drug use in Britain appeared to be increasing at an alarming rate and spreading across the country on an unprecedented scale. An apparent growth in the use of heroin caused particular concern: the number of known heroin addicts rose from just over two thousand in 1977 to more than ten thousand by 1987.[1] Moreover, heroin use was being reported in urban areas throughout the country.[2] This was in contrast to previous decades, when it was thought that drug use was largely confined to London.[3] By 1985 the Conservative government was able to assert that "the misuse of drugs is one of the most worrying problems facing our society today."[4] Growing fears about drug use prompted a flurry of activity from both central and local government, from law enforcement bodies, voluntary organizations, and health professionals.

This article will consider the response to the development of a national heroin "problem" in the 1980s through an examination of the Central Funding Initiative for drug services. The Central Funding Initiative (CFI) was a multi-million-pound program dedicated toward the provision of services for drug users, particularly those in areas away from London and the Southeast. This was, however, more than just a reaction to the spread of drug use to the regions: it was indicative of broader changes within the drugs field and within health and social policy more generally. The CFI was designed to foster a multidisciplinary approach to drug use, providing a range of services, such as residential rehabilitation and street-based counseling, to drug users. This was in contrast to the primarily medically orientated response to drug use in existence since the

The authors wish to thank the Economic and Social Research Council (ESRC) for a project grant (award number RES-000-23-0265) entitled "Drug User Patient Groups, 'User Groups,' and Drug Policy, 1970 to 2004" that has supported this work.

late 1960s, based around out-patient treatment in the National Health Service Drug Dependence Units, a medical response with a much longer history.[5] Through the CFI, less emphasis was placed on treatment alone, suggesting greater attention to the social as well as the medical consequences of drug use. This was to be achieved by involving a wider range of agencies in providing services for drug users. Particular encouragement was given to voluntary organizations because these were regarded as more flexible than statutory bodies, and thus better equipped to respond in new ways to the rapidly developing drug problem.

This article argues that these changes must be understood at two levels. At one level, the history of the Central Funding Initiative could simply be seen as a pioneering development in social policy, illustrative of the wider agenda of the Thatcher government of the 1980s. But at another level, it was also the product of long-standing tensions within drug policy and threw light on the ways in which British health policy was made. Let us briefly survey both these dynamics. Involving the voluntary sector in the provision of services for drug users reflected wider shifts within health and welfare in Britain during the 1980s. The Conservative government, led by Margaret Thatcher, regarded the state as an inefficient and ineffective provider of welfare, and considered its monopoly on the provision of services to have resulted in a culture of passivity and dependence among welfare recipients.[6] The suggested solution to this problem was to "roll back the state"; to reduce the role of central government in the provision of welfare. The "rolling back of the state" was to be achieved in two closely related ways. First, by placing greater emphasis on the involvement of voluntary organizations in the delivery of health and social services, and second, by creating a "market" in welfare, allowing statutory and nonstatutory bodies to bid for contracts to provide specific services.[7] In both these developments the role of the voluntary sector was crucial. Not only was the voluntary sector regarded as being more responsive, more innovative, and more cost-effective than the statutory sector, but it was also thought to be able to reduce reliance on the state through the "invigorating" experience of self-help and community care.[8] However, there was a paradox in these changes, as social policy commentators were quick to point out: increased statutory funding of the voluntary sector tied this more closely to the state than before, leading some to point to the rise of a new state-funded voluntary sector.[9]

Setting the CFI and the provision of services for drug users in this context provides a window onto these broader changes, but there were also more drug-policy-specific reasons for the Initiative. The CFI was the product of growing concern about drug use and its spread across the country. Pressure for action illustrated the importance of new forces in drug policy, such as the voluntary sector and expert advisory committees, forces that typified new definitions of drug use in society. These new forces were to some extent opposed to the dominant medical and psychiatric response to drug use, but the genesis and implementation of the Initiative also illus-trated the power of the medical civil service, a long-standing tendency within British health policy. It is argued, therefore, that the CFI was the product of micro and macro forces, reflecting both specific tensions within the drugs field and the wider move to "roll back the state." In order to tease out these different factors, this article will begin by looking at the develop-ment of the heroin problem in Britain, moving on to examine how this problem came to be recognized, how the CFI responded to it, and, finally, making sense of this response by relating it both to the general changes within welfare in this period and to a specific period of crisis in drug policy.

Developing a Problem

The use of illegal drugs in Britain was not an entirely new phenomenon, but during the 1980s drug use, and the use of heroin in particular, came to dominate popular and political agendas as never before. This was due (at least in part) to a significant change in the size and scale of drug use. Although accurate figures for drug use are notoriously difficult to obtain, some indication of the number of drug users can be gleaned from the Home Office Addicts Index. The Index, established in 1934, was a record of the names of addicts known to the Home Office, based on information derived from police inspections of pharmacists' records and notifications of addiction by doctors.[10] There had been a steady increase in the number of known addicts since the early 1960s, but the total number of cases largely remained under 2,000 until the late 1970s. From 1977 onward, the num-ber of known addicts rose from 2,016 in 1977 to 2,402 in 1978 and 2,666 in 1979. This trend persisted into the 1980s: between 1980 and 1981 the number of notified addicts increased by almost a thousand, a 44 percent increase.[11] Notifications to the Home Office continued to rise throughout the decade, so that by 1987 there were 10,389 known addicts.[12] Despite better reporting of addiction, these figures were thought to be a significant underestimate.[13] The "real" number of drug users was much debated and various multipliers based on epidemiological indicators were brought into play. Some commentators argued that it was quite possible that there were as many as 100,000 heroin addicts in Britain by the end of the 1980s.[14]

In addition to a numerical increase, drug use appeared to be spreading across the country. Before this period the "British drug problem" could perhaps more accurately be described as the "London drug problem," with very few drug users to be found away from the capital. By the end of the 1970s, it was clear that this was no longer the case. Lord Denbigh, in a speech to the House of Lords on drug addiction in 1979, stated that over the past seven years there had been a 127 percent increase in the number of known addicts residing outside the London area.[15] Between 1978 and 1981, most regions saw incidences of addiction double, and a number of studies identified significant heroin use in places such as Merseyside, Manchester, and Glasgow.[16] For the authors of one of those studies, it was clear that this was a "new phenomenon."[17]

This new phenomenon has usually been explained in terms of supply and demand. During the 1960s and early 1970s, most of the heroin used by addicts was legally produced and prescribed, if illegally traded, between users. As the drug could be obtained on prescription from licensed medical practitioners, there was virtually no black market in heroin. This changed dramatically in the late 1970s. Most commentators point to an influx of heroin into Britain following the Iranian Revolution in 1979.[18] The amount of illicit heroin seized by police and customs, likely to represent just a fraction of the total smuggled into the UK, rose considerably. The authorities seized just 3 kilograms of heroin in 1973, compared to 93 kilograms in 1981.[19] What is more, in real terms, the price of black-market heroin fell by as much as 25 percent between 1980 and 1983.[20] Significantly, most of this heroin was so-called "brown" heroin, particularly well suited to smoking rather than injecting. This was important, as studies suggested that potential users who might be put off heroin by the danger and stigma attached to injection would feel less reluctant to try the drug if they could smoke it. By the mid-1980s, it was clear that there was a plentiful supply of relatively cheap, illegally produced and distributed heroin to be found in Britain.[21]

Explaining the corresponding rise in demand is much more difficult and remains a sensitive and complex issue. Contemporary interpretations have been characterized by the sociologist Susanne MacGregor as being either of the "Right" or the "Left." Those on the Right usually emphasized the immorality of young drug users and their further corruption by evil drug "pushers." In contrast, those on the Left argued that there was a link between drug use and growing deprivation and unemployment.[22] This was consistently denied by the Conservative government: the Home Office minister in charge of drug policy, David Mellor, told the House of Commons in 1986 that "no link between the taking of drugs and unemployment has been established. The taking of drugs," he continued "is much more closely linked to pressure from friends and curiosity."[23] It is difficult to deny, however, that the 1980s were a time of considerable social, political, and economic turmoil in Britain. Unemployment was high throughout the decade, reaching over 3 million in 1982. Furthermore, unemployment was particularly high among young people in urban areas hit hard by the restructuring of the economy, such as the North East, North West, and industrial areas of Scotland, the very same regions that began to experience extensive drug use for the first time.[24] A possible connection between drug use and deprivation has become less controversial in recent years, with research in the United States, Britain, and other parts of Europe pointing to a strong association between drug use and the social environment, but the wider debate on the causation of drug use continues.[25] Indeed, caution must be exercised when making links between drugs and deprivation, as drug use in this period developed into a much wider social phenomenon. While drug use could undoubtedly be found in areas of high unemployment, it also could be found in areas of relative affluence. Journalist Marek Kohn detailed media responses to drug use in the 1980s and found that it was often portrayed as a problem for people "who live on big estates—country ones and council ones."[26]

Irrespective of the cause of the rise in drug use during the early 1980s, what was beyond doubt was that existing services were unable to cope with the increased number of drug users and their widening geographical spread. Since 1968, treatment for drug addiction was largely to be found in the Drug Dependence Units or DDUs, staffed by consultant psychiatrists: these units had replaced previous general-practitioner involvement in the treatment of drug users.[27] By the 1980s, treatment usually involved the prescription of an opiate drug (typically oral methadone, but some psychiatrists were licensed to prescribe heroin to addicts) on a reducing basis, resulting in detoxification.[28] Following withdrawal from drugs, ex-users could seek residential rehabilitation in a variety of facilities run by voluntary organizations. Voluntary agencies also ran a handful of street-based centers, offering counseling and legal advice to drug users.[29] These services, however, were not uniformly dispersed around the country. Most DDUs were to be found in the Thames area (the region surrounding London). So too were the majority of advice and counseling services and residential rehabilitation facilities.[30] In the regions, services were often limited to a handful of interested psychiatrists and general practitioners. A Sheffield-based psychiatrist stated in an interview that "in the seventies our nearest, if you like, tertiary [specialist] unit was in Nottingham [a town approximately 45 miles away]. And in the time I worked in Sheffield I think I managed to get two people admitted there from Sheffield."[31] Even in London, where many of the DDUs were located, services were increasingly overburdened by the growing numbers of addicts seeking treatment, resulting in long waiting lists.[32]

Moreover, there was evidence to suggest that the DDUs were seeing a declining proportion of drug users. A change in treatment policy had occurred in the 1970s replacing maintenance (long-term prescription of opiate drugs) policies with those based on abstinence: it was this development and the forces behind it that were also an important dynamic for the CFI. From the changes of 1968 onward, heroin addiction had been a formally notifiable condition: doctors were required to notify the Home Office when they came into contact with an addict patient, although many had been notifying informally for many years before that.[33] Most notifications came initially from doctors working in prisons and at DDUs: in 1970, 46 percent of notifications of heroin addiction came from DDUs, 48 percent from prison medical officers, and just six percent from general practitioners (GPs). By 1981 the proportion of notifications from DDUs had fallen to 36 percent and notifications by prison medical officers to 16 percent, whereas notifications by GPs had risen to 48 percent of the total.[34] It would seem that drug users were increasingly deserting the DDUs. In part this was because of changing patterns of drug use with a move away from the exclusive use of heroin toward more "polydrug" use, with users taking a range of drugs, including heroin, opiate substitutes, and barbiturates. Yet, at DDUs, according to *The Lancet*, there was "a near total preoccupation with opiate dependence."[35] A major reason was also that, by the 1980s, the main treatment offered by DDUs was a rapidly reducing course of oral methadone, with an ultimate focus on abstinence, something many addicts did not find acceptable. This change in policy came not from government, which took little interest in drug policy at the political level, but from the group of psychiatrists who ran the London DDUs. They had adopted a consensual policy in order to prevent the "silting up" of the clinics with long-term maintenance cases and also as a means of regulating supply.[36] For these reasons, drug services established in the late 1960s were clearly not able to cope with the changing nature of the drug problem in the 1980s.

Recognizing the Problem: The New Forces in Drug Policy

Throughout the 1970s, drugs had not been a political issue or even a matter of great political interest. The response was a matter of consensus rather than one of party political division. It was not politics initially that put the matter on the policy agenda but rather the new forces emergent in drug policy, the new "policy community" of the 1980s. A new "policy community" began to form within the drugs field. There was a shift from a primarily medically orientated policy community to one that included voluntary organizations, researchers, civil servants, and politicians.[37] Initially it was the voluntary sector that raised questions about treatment policy. Voluntary agencies working in the drugs field had been represented since the early 1970s by the umbrella group Standing Conference on Drug Abuse (SCODA, founded in 1973). SCODA had established its power networks in the course of that decade: it lobbied government for changes in drug policy through the formation of close relationships with key civil servants, membership of advisory bodies such as the Advisory Council on Drug Misuse (ACMD), and by establishing the All-Party Parliamentary Working Group on Drug Misuse.[38] From the late 1970s onward, SCODA began to report increasing contact with people from all over the country who were seeking help with drug problems but were unable to find local services.[39] SCODA was also critical of official statistics on drug use, arguing that the problem was much bigger than the government realized as "the experience of many voluntary organizations is that a high proportion of their client group remains un-notified and in consequence, officially 'unknown.'"[40] By the early 1980s, SCODA was reporting that while the number of drug users continued to grow, services had failed to expand, which resulted in additional pressure on existing facilities. This led the body to call for intervention from central government, arguing in its annual report in 1981 that "ad hoc responses at a local level are inadequate at a time when all the indices of drug problems show a rapid rise and when there is a dearth of specialist services in many parts of the country. Without a central government initiative which includes central financing, there can be little hope that a suitable pattern and range of services can be developed."[41]

SCODA was not the only body calling for greater involvement from central government. The role of the Advisory Council on the Misuse of Drugs (ACMD) was crucial. The council, originally convened in 1966 as the Advisory Committee on Drug Dependence, was established in 1971 as part of the changes in policy enshrined in the Misuse of Drugs Act. It was representative of a new style of expert committee set up in the 1970s in the health field and was to advise the government "on measures to prevent and deal with the social problems arising from the misuse of drugs."[42] Its membership illustrated the widening "policy community" around the drugs issue, with individuals from a wide range of fields connected with drug use, such as psychiatrists, nurses, social workers, probation officers, and voluntary agencies. The expert committee was an important instigator of new approaches in the drugs field, in particular through its influential report on Treatment and Rehabilitation, published in 1982. This report had a long gestation. In 1975 the ACMD created a working group to review treatment and rehabilitation services for drug users. The working group's interim report, published in 1977, did express some concern that the number of drug users appeared to be rising and that treatment services might not be equipped to cope with such an increase, but the group felt that "much can be achieved towards the establishment, at little or no additional cost, of the necessary facilities for the treatment of drug-misusers by the wise deployment of existing resources."[43] This assertion did not convince everyone. A civil servant asked to comment on the resource implications of the interim report remarked that "it will be a difficult task to persuade health authorities to provide additional resources or indeed maintain the present level, in the current economic climate, for this small group of patients." He suspected that "you will probably have to offer the carrot of special funding to achieve anything new."[44]

This was a prescient statement. By 1979 it was increasingly clear to the ACMD that more resources would be needed to fund drug services. Once more, pressure came from the voluntary sector. David Turner, coordinator of SCODA and a member of the ACMD, told the council that the burgeoning market in illicit drugs and the growth of drug use outside London meant that "treatment services must be expanded to cope with the impending explosion of demand." For Turner, it was essential that the ACMD's final report "should explore areas of funding in relation to providing new services and to improving the options available to existing ones."[45] Turner's was not a lone voice. Dr. Anthony Thorley, a consultant psychiatrist at Newcastle Teaching Hospital, felt that "without central funding the grass roots services would always live a hand to mouth existence as drug misusers were a stigmatised section of society."[46] This view was reflected in the final report, "Treatment and Rehabilitation," published in 1982. The ACMD noted that the stigma attached to drug addiction made funding services for drug users a low priority when allocating resources. To combat this, the report recommended that "there should be increased funding, direct from central government, possibly by way of pump-priming grants."[47] This, it was hoped, would lead to the development of multidisciplinary services for drug users in every region.

The key facilitator of the new approach within government was, ironically, a doctor. Dr. Dorothy Black, senior medical officer at the DHSS with responsibility for drug policy, was a central figure in the stimulation and implementation of the new policy.[48] Black began work at the DHSS in 1981, but had previously been a psychiatrist involved in the treatment of drug users in a Northern city. She brought with her to the DHSS the knowledge that the drug problem had already spread beyond London, and also a sense that local authorities had little interest in funding services for drug users. During her time in the North, she had also set up a local council on drugs and had worked with the voluntary sector.[49] Moreover, Black's appointment was itself a tacit recognition that drug use was becoming a problem. Previously, drugs and alcohol had been dealt with together by the DHSS, with the greater emphasis placed on alcohol policy. A senior civil servant commented that by 1982 "people were beginning to pay more attention, partly because it was felt that there was an increasing number of people using drugs, which was supported by the figures of the Home Office Index, and so it was decided that something must be done."[50] Behind this rational justification of change also lay a two-pronged strategy that sought to undermine the power of the London psychiatrists. First, to develop a variety of treatment approaches, prescribing as well as nonprescribing, and second, to enhance services outside London.[51]

Doing Something about the Problem: The Central Funding Initiative

On December 1, 1982, the Secretary of State for Social Services, Norman Fowler, whose political support was important for the changes in drug policy, announced that £2 million would be made available for grants to local authorities and voluntary bodies to provide services for drug users in England.[52] Similar schemes were to be set up in Scotland and Wales.[53] Initially, the Central Funding Initiative was designed to provide £6 million over three years, but the program was extended in January 1986, partly in response to the discovery of HIV/AIDS among injecting drug users. Under the initiative, a total of £17.5 million was awarded to both statutory and voluntary bodies between 1983 and 1989.[54] The scheme operated by setting aside "earmarked" funds exclusively for drug services that local authorities and voluntary groups could bid for by applying to the DHSS for a grant. Most funding from central to local government was not usually directed toward a specific aim, but, according to Dorothy Black, it was felt that the only way local authorities could be persuaded to do anything about drug use was to provide funding.[55] As MacGregor and Ettore noted, "Health Authorities find it difficult to put services for drug misusers ahead of those for, say, kidney transplants or old people."[56] What was also significant about the CFI was the way funds were issued. Grants were made on a pump-priming basis: agencies in receipt of a grant were expected to find alternative sources of funding once this came to an end. For voluntary agencies, this meant securing the support of the relevant local authority at the time of application.[57] This was designed to ensure that when the fixed period of central funding finished, services would not disappear.[58]

The CFI had four stated objectives: first, to provide regional and local assessments of the drug problem; second, to improve awareness of the problems related to drug "misuse" and the ability of people working in this area to help; third, to improve links between health services provision and community provision; and, finally, to improve the effectiveness of services and their value for the money.[59] Those involved in the initiative remembered the intensive way in which they operated. A senior civil servant recalled that "I used to be there until 8, 9 o'clock reading through these things [applications]" but also that all the proposals were "read by all the professionals in the drug policy group, which were myself, my nursing colleague, and by one of the administrative officers, and we then came to a consensus about what we could fund."[60]

It was clear from the outset that the CFI was designed to improve services for drug users throughout the nation. Under-secretary of State for Health and Social Security, John Patten, told a committee of MPs examining the nature of drug services in 1985 that "the concentration of facilities for drug abuse has been in London and the South East, but it is a growing problem in other parts of the country and it would be wrong if we did not spread these resources around the country."[61] The pattern of grants made supported this. A total of 188 grants were made under the CFI between 1983 and 1989, and, as Patten remarked, "places north of London will not have cause to complain" about the allocation of money.[62] Indeed, Chris Smith, MP for Islington and Finsbury, asserted that CFI funds had "largely bypassed London," an allegation quickly quashed by the government and not borne out by the actual allocation of resources. All of the fourteen Regional Health Authorities received some funds, although not equally. Areas thought to have the most extensive drug use (the Thames region and Merseyside) received the most money. The team of researchers employed to assess the effectiveness of the CFI concluded that "the allocation exercise seems to have been successful in targeting areas of need."[63] London did not necessarily lose out in terms of the funding allocation (45 percent of the grants were awarded to projects in the Thames region); rather it was a case of the regions gaining funding for service provision where there had been none before.

Yet the CFI did, to some extent, also mark the lessening of the capital's influence on the general shape and direction of drug services. Prior to the CFI, drug policy and provision had been dominated by the Drug Dependence Units. Of the 22 DDUs nationwide, 16 were located in the Thames region, most of these in the London teaching hospitals.[64] As these were run by specialist psychiatrists, the DDUs could be seen as being representative of a medical approach to drug use.[65] But as the number of drug users increased during the 1980s and the effects of drug use were felt within society on a larger scale, questions were raised about medicine's dominant role in drug policy.[66] This was exemplified by a change in the terms utilized to describe drug users from "addicts" in the 1960s to "problem drug takers" in the 1980s.[67] "Problem drug takers" appeared to require the help and support of a much wider range of agencies than "addicts." A senior civil servant remarked that the DHSS view at this time was that DDUs should give "further thought to the sort of treatment programme they should approach; that it shouldn't just be an entirely medical, clinical one."[68] This resulted in an increasingly multidisciplinary approach to drug use, in contrast to the medically orientated London-based DDUs.[69]

The type of services supported by the CFI both exemplified and accelerated these trends. Almost half (46 percent) of CFI funds went to community-based walk-in centers; 20 percent to multidisciplinary community drug teams; and 16 percent to residential rehabilitation facilities, leaving just 18 percent of funds for DDUs and hospital-based services.[70] After the CFI, drug services, according to the team of researchers tasked with assessing its impact, could best be described as "pluralistic."[71] An important aspect of this pluralism was the role played by voluntary organizations. Voluntary groups had been involved in caring for drug users since the 1960s and some had received funding from the DHSS. Most of this funding, in line with more general support for nonstatutory groups in the health field, was provided under Section 64 of the Public Health Services and Public Health Act of 1968 and largely confined to headquarters administrative expenses for voluntary bodies working on a national basis.[72] Both SCODA and the Institute for the Study of Drug Dependence, a drugs information service and specialist library, received funding in this manner.[73] Smaller, local groups tended to receive funds on an ad hoc basis or from local authorities, such as the London Boroughs Association.[74] Most agencies, however, were chronically underfunded. The ACMD, noted that "the non-statutory agencies involved in treatment and rehabilitation rely on an insecure combination of local and central government funding and exist under the constant threat of financial collapse."[75]

Providing central funds for voluntary organizations in order to prevent them from disappearing was not the sole reason for opening up the

Central Funding Initiative to nonstatutory groups. A DHSS circular informing regional authorities of the introduction of the CFI stated that its purpose was "not to remove from statutory authorities the responsibility for providing services and training but, by making additional funds available to them and to voluntary organizations, to remedy more rapidly than would otherwise have been possible, the inadequacy of the network of services for people with drug related problems."[76] Fostering the participation of voluntary organizations was vital because, as Patten told MPs, there was a realization that "the problem is not necessarily going to be ameliorated and controlled . . . by action within the National Health Service alone." Moreover, "A very great deal of expertise, in terms of prevention and counselling, is in the voluntary sector, not in the National Health Service."[77] Yet, nonstatutory groups did not just provide expertise: there was a feeling among DHSS officials that voluntary organizations offered something statutory authorities could not. A senior civil servant asserted that voluntary groups "could be more flexible in what they did," that as they "were not tied to a specific service approach . . . they were more willing to initiate different types of services."[78] The CFI, by offering substantial funding to voluntary organizations, was designed to make use of this. Even so, a senior civil servant remarked that "we were quite surprised that we got so many applications from the voluntary sector"; clearly developments on the ground had been somewhat invisible at the central policy level.[79] Yet once the DHSS was aware of the extent of voluntary sector involvement in the field, a clear commitment was made to enhancing its role in drug service provision. This can be seen in the grants made under the CFI: of the 188 grants issued, 58 percent went to statutory organizations and 42 percent to nonstatutory groups.[80] Such significant support for voluntary organizations cannot be explained by necessity alone: this must be related to a much broader strategy for involving the nonstatutory sector in health and social service provision.

The House of Commons Social Services Committee tasked with investigating drug "misuse" in 1985 were supportive of a greater role for voluntary organizations in drug services, but were concerned about the short-term nature of pump-priming grants, and recommended that "adequate funding [be] guaranteed for a number of years." Furthermore, although most witnesses to the Social Services Committee welcomed the CFI, some were concerned that "it will produce a pattern of services which is haphazard and not truly reflective of need."[81]

This criticism resulted in the DHSS commissioning a team, led by Susanne MacGregor, to evaluate the CFI.[82] The evaluation of policy initiatives was becoming increasingly valued by the DHSS. Other dedicated funding schemes run by the department were also assessed by professional researchers, with the evaluation usually being commissioned at the beginning of the initiative.[83] A DHSS official noted in a letter to MacGregor: "Obviously an evaluation of the initiative as a whole should have been mounted at the beginning; for various reasons it wasn't but the customers feel that there is a useful exercise that can still be done."[84] While the department felt that an evaluation would be useful for "both accountability purposes and for general guidance on the further development of services for service planners and policy makers," it might also be suggested that it was required in order to justify policy change and significant expenditure on a heavily stigmatized group.[85] But the strategy also marked the rise of the role of evidence in health policy and a developing role for research: it exemplified trends that were to develop later in the 1980s through the directed funding for AIDS and the NHS Research and Development initiative.[86]

Making Sense of the Problem:
The CFI and Drug Services in Context

In many ways, the Central Funding Initiative for drug services represents a microcosm of key aspects of Conservative welfare policy in this period. The term "initiative" was a particular favorite of the Thatcher administration. Numerous "initiatives" were launched to tackle a range of social issues, particularly in the inner cities. Urban development grants, for example, were designed to foster regeneration by using public funds to pump-prime development in areas such as the London Docklands and Merseyside. Central to these policies was the notion of "partnership" with private companies and voluntary organizations, which would be expected to support projects in the long term.[87] In the health field, "initiative" had a particular meaning. From 1982 onward a number of central funding initiatives were launched in areas where the government wanted to raise standards. Alongside the drug users initiative, there were CFIs to provide improved services for children under five years old, better services for mentally ill elderly people, enhanced services for mentally disabled children, and more general initiatives such as Opportunities for Volunteering and Helping the Community to Care.[88] A DHSS official noted that "the funding of schemes is deliberately limited in duration to preserve their development and catalyst role. They are not intended as a prolonged substitute for local funding." Health and local authorities were expected to find the money for continuing schemes from within their regular sources of funding, and voluntary bodies were required to continue raising their own funds.[89]

Such a scheme cast central government in the role of initiator of new services rather than its long-term funder. The central funding initiatives thus encapsulated a key aspect of the Thatcherite policy of "rolling back the state," reducing direct statutory involvement in welfare provision by changing the function of the state from that of provider to manager, but through a command-and-control model.[90] This transition was later confirmed through the NHS Care and Community Act in 1990. The act created an internal market within health and social care by establishing a divide between the "purchasers" of services and the "providers." Local authorities, for example, were able to "purchase" a particular service, such as a needle exchange for intravenous drug users, from a local "provider." The "provider" could be a statutory, voluntary, or private organization; these providers were expected to "compete" within the internal market for the custom of the "purchaser." Competition, it was argued, would make services more cost-effective and responsive to consumer demand.[91]

The creation of the internal market, it has been argued, helped to replace "welfare statism" with "welfare pluralism" as a range of groups and organizations took on functions previously performed by the state.[92] Within what Jane Lewis has called the "mixed economy of care," particular significance was placed on the part played by voluntary organizations.[93] The voluntary sector was regarded as being more flexible than the statutory sector and, crucially, more able to enhance citizen participation.[94] Reliance on the state could be further reduced as individuals would be afforded the "invigorating" experience of self-help and community care.[95] Of course there is a paradox here—as statutory support for voluntary organizations increased, and was formalized during the 1990s with the introduction of contracts between purchasers and providers, elements of what was distinctive about the voluntary, as opposed to the statutory, sector could be seen to have diminished.[96] Susanne MacGregor and Ben Pimlott asserted that some organizations were transformed into "*de facto* agencies of the state, which financed them and indirectly determined their policy."[97] As Rodney Lowe has remarked in relation to the creation of the internal market more generally, this did not automatically result in a reduction of statutory funding for welfare and cannot have been said to have "rolled back the state." Yet, he is forced to conclude that the internal market was Thatcher's major legacy in social policy.[98] A crucial part of that legacy was in creating much closer relationships between voluntarism and the state.

Conclusion

The Central Funding Initiative for drug users thus needs to be understood in relation to two crises in the early 1980s, one specifically in drug policy and one more generally in the political perception of the role of state provision in social policy. The expanding drug problem, the inadequacy of existing services (especially in the regions), and a desire to shift these services away from a purely medical or psychiatric approach to drug use were clearly the key factors in the establishment of a dedicated funding program for drug services, but the shape that this took was influenced by broader changes in the nature of the welfare state in Britain.

At the level of drug policy, the CFI highlighted the existence of a new "policy community," within which the power of the voluntary sector was exerted through the doctor civil servant, an alliance that was to develop over the following decades. The most obvious immediate consequence of the CFI was to create a much more diverse and extensive network of services for drug users throughout Britain than had previously existed. Services were increasingly multidisciplinary rather than just medical in nature, facilitating the development of a broader understanding of drug use and its social implications. The CFI's support for voluntary organizations and community-based services was particularly significant: these services came to play a key role in the response to the next crisis of the 1980s, the advent of HIV/AIDS and its spread among drug users. As Black stated at a conference in 1989, AIDS was a "golden opportunity to get it right for the first time" and the spread of syringe exchange was an additional stimulus to a national system that bypassed the DDUs. Had the CFI not existed, the basis for this extension of services would not have existed.[99] Many voluntary groups were leading proponents of the harm-minimization approach to drug use that achieved official sanction following the ACMD's report on AIDS and drug misuse in 1988.[100] In a context where AIDS was viewed as a greater threat to public health than drug use, the voice of the drug user in determining the nature of services was accorded greater weight.

The CFI was, therefore, undoubtedly a product of a specific crisis—the developing drug problem in the 1980s—but it also exemplified broader changes in health and welfare policy. Coming as it did, just before the establishment of the internal market, the CFI prefigured many of its key aspects: central government as the funder but not the provider of services, the increased devolution to local authorities as purchasers of services, and the growing use of nonstatutory organizations in service provision. Furthermore, in the role it gave to research and evaluation, the CFI was also a harbinger of evidence-based arguments within policy that were to become important in the 1990s and the early twenty-first century. The CFI was not just an innovative initiative for drug policy: it was a pilot for policy initiatives much more broadly.

It is no surprise, therefore, that the CFI also exemplified some of the inherent contradictions within health and welfare policy in this period. On the one hand, the CFI's encouragement of voluntary organizations, and the devolution of responsibility for the continued success of these groups to local authorities, appeared to be a reduction of the role played by central government in the organization of drug services. Yet, on the other hand, funding for these services was decided upon centrally, maintaining a crucial role for the DHSS in determining the general shape and direction of drug policy. This is analogous to what has been described as the "command-and-control" tendencies of the Thatcher administration, where the rhetoric of enhancing freedom and choice actually masked a significant degree of centralization. As our analysis of the CFI and drug policy in the 1980s has demonstrated, the state was not so much "rolled back" in this period as "rolled in," forming a constituent part of an increasingly diverse mix of welfare providers. It is a legacy that lives on.

London School of Hygiene and Tropical Medicine
University of London

Notes

1. Precise figures are 1977, 2,016; 1987, 10,389. Home Office, *Statistics of Drug Addicts Notified to the Home Office*, 1988 (London, 1989).
2. Advisory Council on the Misuse of Drugs (ACMD), *Treatment and Rehabilitation* (London, 1982), 25.
3. Ministry of Health, *Drug Addiction: Report of the Second Interdepartmental Committee* (London, 1964), 8.
4. Home Office, *Tackling Drug Misuse: A Summary of the Government's Strategy* (London, 1985), foreword.
5. V. Berridge, "The 'British System' and Its History: Myth and Reality," in J. Strang and M. Gossop, eds., *Heroin Addiction and the British System. Volume 1, Origins and Evolution* (London, 2005), 7–16.
6. G. Finlayson, *Citizen, State, and Social Welfare in Britain, 1830–1990* (Oxford, 1994), 357–60.
7. N. Deakin, "The Perils of Partnership: The Voluntary Sector and the State, 1945–1992," in J. Davis Smith, C. Rochester, and R. Hedley, eds., *An Introduction to the Voluntary Sector* (London, 1995), 40-65; 54–62; J. Kendall and J. and M. Knapp, *The Voluntary Sector in the United Kingdom* (Manchester, 1996), 201–5; J. Lewis, "Developing the Mixed Economy of Care: Emerging Issues for Voluntary Organisations," *Journal of Social Policy* 22, no. 2 (1993): 173–92.
8. For an overview of welfare policy under Thatcher, see R. Lowe, *The Welfare State in Britain Since 1945*, 3d ed. (Basingstoke, 2005), 317–27, 350–57.

9. S. MacGregor and B. Pimlott, "Action and Inaction in the Cities," in S. MacGregor and B. Pimlott, *Tackling the Inner Cities: The 1980s Reviewed, Prospects for the 1990s* (Oxford, 1990), 9. Although of course state funding of the voluntary sector was nothing new, see V. Berridge, "New Social Movement or Government-funded Voluntary Sector? ASH (Action on Smoking and Health) Science and Anti-tobacco Activism in the 1970s," in M. Pelling and S. Mandelbrote, eds., *The Practice of Reform in Health, Medicine, and Science, 1500–2000: Essays for Charles Webster* (London, 2005), 333–48.

10. H. B. Spear, *Heroin Addiction Care and Control: The British System, 1916–1984* (London, 2002), 41–42.

11. Home Office, *Statistics of Drug Addicts Notified to the Home Office, United Kingdom, 1988* (London, 1989).

12. Ibid.

13. G. Stimson, "British Drug Policies in the 1980s: A Preliminary Analysis and Suggestions for Research," in V. Berridge, ed., *Drugs Research and Policy in Britain: A Review of the 1980s* (Aldershot, 1990), 260–81; and J. Mott, "Notification and the Home Office," in Strang and Gossop, ed., *Heroin Addiction and Drug Policy*, 271–91; 287.

14. S. MacGregor, "The Public Debate in the 1980s," in S. MacGregor, ed., *Drugs and British Society: Responses to a Social Problem in the 1980s* (London, 1989), 1–19; 3.

15. *The Hansard Journal of Parliamentary Debates: Lords*, 30 October 1979, 355.

16. For a breakdown in regional notifications, see ACMD, *Treatment and Rehabilitation*, 121–27.

17. H. Parker, R. Newcombe, and K. Bakx, "The New Heroin Users: Prevalence and Characteristics in Wirral, Merseyside," *British Journal of Addiction* (1987): 82, 147–57; 147.

18. R. Davenport-Hines, *The Pursuit of Oblivion: A Global History of Narcotics, 1500–2000* (London, 2001), 364; R. Power, "Drug Trends since 1968," in Strang and Gossop, eds., *Heroin Addiction and Drug Policy*, 27–41; 34–35.

19. ACMD, *Treatment and Rehabilitation*, 130.

20. P. Griffiths, M. Gossop, and J. Strang, "Chasing the Dragon: The Development of Heroin Smoking in the United Kingdom," in Strang and Gossop, eds., *Heroin Addiction and Drug Policy*, 121–33; 124.

21. G. Stimson, "The War on Heroin: British Policy and the International Trade in Illicit Drugs," in N. Dorn and N. South, eds., *A Land Fit for Heroin? Drug Policies, Prevention, and Practice* (Basingstoke, 1987), 35–61; 39–41; R. Lewis, "Flexible Hierarchies and Dynamic Disorder: The Trading and Distribution of Illicit Heroin in Britain and Europe, 1970–1990," in Strang and Gossop, *Heroin Addiction and Drug Policy*, 42–65; Spear, Heroin Addiction Care and Control, 255–74.

22. MacGregor, "The Public Debate in the 1980s," 3. The key contemporary paper detailing the link with unemployment was D. F. Peck and M. A. Plant, "Unemployment and Illegal Drug Use: Concordant Evidence from a Prospective Study and National Trends," *British Medical Journal* 293 (11 October 1986).

23. *Hansard Journal of Political Debates: House of Commons*, vol. 91 (1985–86), p. 296, col. 568.

24. Lowe, *The Welfare State in Britain*, 325; J. Harris, "Tradition and Transformation: Society and Civil Society in Britain, 1945–2000," in K. Burk, ed., *The British Isles Since 1945* (Oxford, 2003), 91–125; 112.

25. For an overview of the debate on deprivation and drug use, see G. Pearson and M. Gilman, "Drug Epidemics in Space and Time: Local Diversity, Subcultures, and Social Exclusion," in Strang and Gossop, *Heroin Addiction and the British System*, 1:109–14.

26. M. Kohn, *Narcomania: On Heroin* (London, 1987), 114.

27. A. Mold, "The 'British System' of Heroin Addiction Treatment and the Opening of the Drug Dependence Units, 1965–1970,' *Social History of Medicine* 17, no. 3 (2004): 501–17.

28. On treatment methods, see A. Mold, "Dynamic Dualities: The British System of Heroin Addiction Treatment, 1965–1987" (Ph.D. thesis, University of Birmingham, 2004).

29. N. Dorn and N. South, *Helping Drug Users* (London, 1985); A. Mold, "The Welfare Branch of the Alternative Society? The Work of Drug Voluntary Organisation Release, 1967–1978," *Twentieth Century British History* 17, no. 1 (2006): 50–73.

30. S. MacGregor, B. Ettorre, R. Coomber, A. Crosier, and H. Lodge, *Drug Services in England and the Impact of the Central Funding Initiative* (London, 1991), 6, 28.

31. Interview conducted by authors with a Sheffield-based psychiatrist, 2 May 2006.

32. House of Commons Social Services Committee, *Misuse of Drugs*, liii; J. Love and M. Gossop, "The Processes of Referral and Disposal within a London Drug Dependence Clinic," *British Journal of Addiction* 80 (1985): 435–40; 438.

33. Mold, "The 'British System,'" 506, 509.

34. ACMD, *Treatment and Rehabilitation*, 120.

35. "Drug addiction: British System failing," *Lancet* (9 January 1982): 83–84; 83.

36. S. Mars, "Peer Pressure and Imposed Consensus: The Making of the 1984 Guidelines of Good Clinical Practice in the Treatment of Drug Misuse," in V. Berridge, ed., *Making Health Policy: Networks in Research and Policy after 1945* (Amsterdam, 2005), 149-82.

37. V. Berridge, "AIDS and British Drug Policy: Continuity or Change?" in V. Berridge and P. Strong, eds., *AIDS and Contemporary History* (Cambridge, 1993), 135–56; 141.

38. Interview conducted by authors with David Turner, former director of SCODA, 25 February 2005.

39. DrugScope Library, London (hereafter DL), record no. 30658, *SCODA Annual Report, 1977-78*, 2-3.

40. DL 32718, *SCODA Annual Report, 1978–79*, 12.

41. DL 36959, *SCODA Annual Report, 1980–81*, 6.

42. ACMD, *Treatment and Rehabilitation*, 3. For a membership list, see ibid., 87–88.

43. The National Archives, Kew (hereafter TNA), MH 154/1149, letter to Minister for Health from Sir Robert Bradshaw, chairman of the ACMD, 25 June 1977.

44. TNA MH 154/1148, Minutes from M. E. G. Fogden to Mrs. Pearson, 28 February 1977.

45. TNA MH 154/1151, Minutes of the 27th meeting of the ACMD Treatment and Rehabilitation Working Group, 28 June 1979.

46. Ibid.

47. ACMD, *Treatment and Rehabilitation*, 79.

48. Interview conducted by authors with key social science researcher, 10 February 2005.

49. Interview conducted by authors with Dr. Dorothy Black, 2 May 2006.

50. Interview conducted by authors and key civil servant, 2 May 2006.

51. Berridge, "AIDS and British Drug Policy," 141; interview between authors and Professor Gerry Stimson, 17 May 2006.

52. *Hansard Journal of Parliamentary Debates: House of Commons*, vol. 33 (1982–83), p. 704, col. 212.

53. DL 42638, *SCODA Annual Report, 1983–84*, 4.

54. MacGregor et al., *Drug Services in England*.

55. Interview conducted by authors with Dr. Dorothy Black, 2 May 2006.

56. MacGregor and Ettorre, "From Treatment to Rehabilitation," 145.

57. DOHA (Department of Health Archive, Nelson, Lancashire: papers released under the Freedom of Information Act, 2000), OCG/1/1/3, letter from DHSS to all Regional Health Authorities regarding Treatment and Rehabilitation report of the Advisory Council on the Misuse of Drugs (ACMD); Central Funding Initiative (HN (83) 13 LASSAL (83) 1), 25 April 1983, ii.

58. Interview conducted by authors with Dr. Dorothy Black, 2 May 2006.

59. *Hansard Journal of Parliamentary Debates: House of Commons*, vol. 41 (1982–83), p. 806, col. 397.

60. Interview between authors and senior civil servant.

61. House of Commons Social Services Committee report, DHSS evidence, 13 March 1985, 171.

62. MacGregor et al., *Drug Services in England*; House of Commons Social Services Committee report, DHSS evidence, 13 March 1985, 174.

63. MacGregor et al., *Drug Services in England*, 70.

64. Ibid., 28.

65. To some extent DDUs did combine social and medical approaches by aiming to treat and control the drug problem. See Mold, "The 'British System.'"

66. See, for example, Stimson, "British Drug Policies in the 1980s."

67. For an analysis of this, see ibid. For the reports, see Ministry of Health, *Drug Addiction*, and ACMD, *Treatment and Rehabilitation*.

68. Interview conducted by authors with senior civil servant.

69. For a case study of the different approaches adopted at this time by some regional psychiatrists, see J. Strang, "A Model Service: Turning the Generalist on to Drugs," in S. MacGregor, ed., *Drugs and British Society*, 143-69.

70. MacGregor et al., *Drug Services in England*, 45.

71. Ibid., 8.

72. TNA MH 154/433, letter from Mr. J. C. Eversfield, DHSS to Mr. Platten, Town Clerk London Borough of Enfield, 20 December 1971.

73. For SCODA, see TNA MH 154/1192, "Future Developments of the Standing Conference on Drug Abuse" (SCODA) and SCODA annual reports in DrugScope Library; for ISDD, see TNA FD 23/1949, Institute for the Study of Drug Dependence: proposal to set up the Institute, 1967-76, and ISDD annual reports in DrugScope Library.

74. TNA MH 154/430, "Heroin Addiction: London Boroughs Association"; working party reports on rehabilitation, 1968-74.

75. ACMD, *Treatment and Rehabilitation*, 77.

76. DOHA (Department of Health Archive, Nelson, Lancashire) OCG/1/1/3, letter from DHSS to all Regional Health Authorities regarding Treatment and Rehabilitation report of the Advisory Council on the Misuse of Drugs (ACMD); Central Funding Initiative, (HN (83) 13 LASSAL (83) 1), 25 April 1983, 1.

77. DHSS evidence of House of Commons Social Services Committee, 170.

78. Interview conducted by authors with senior civil servant.

79. Ibid.

80. MacGregor et al., *Drug Services in England*, 71-74.

81. House of Commons Social Services Committee, *The Misuse of Drugs*, liii, xlvii.

82. Interview between authors and Susanne MacGregor.

83. DOHA, JR/01980565/V0001A, paper for discussion at drugs client team meeting on research project on CFI, 31 October 1985.

84. DOHA, JR/01980565/V0001A, letter from Anne Kauder, Office of the Chief Scientist, DHSS to Susanne MacGregor, 17 January 1986.

85. DOHA, JR/01980565/V0001A, paper for discussion at drugs client team meeting on research project on CFI, 31 October 1985.

86. N. Black, "The NHS Research and Development Programme: The First Five Years, 1991-6," seminar paper at London School of Hygiene and Tropical Medicine, 21 January 1997.

87. On urban initiatives, see MacGregor and Pimlott, "Action and Inaction in the Cities."

88. DOHA, DAC/0007/V0004, note on Central Initiatives by John H. James, 30 April 1986; DOHA, DAC/0026/V001, memorandum from D. C. Nye to Mr. Alderman, Miss Davies, Mr. Hillier, Mr. Lutterloch, Mr. Pagan, and Mr. Woolley, regarding new initiatives, 14 December 1983.

89. DOHA, DAC/0007/V0004, note on Central Initiatives by John H. James, 30 April 1986.

90. On changes in the welfare state in this period, see Lowe, *The Welfare State*, 317-27.

91. Ibid., 325-26.

92. M. Harris, C. Rochester, and P. Halfpenny, "Voluntary Organisations and Social Policy: Twenty Years of Change," in M. Harris and C. Rochester, eds., *Voluntary Organisations and Social Policy in Britain: Perspectives on Change and Choice* (Basingstoke, 2001), 3.

93. J. Lewis, "Developing the Mixed Economy of Care: Emerging Issues for Voluntary Organisations," *Journal of Social Policy* 22, no. 2 (1993): 173-92.

94. Kendall and Knapp, *The Voluntary Sector in the UK*, 138; Deakin, "The Perils of Partnership," 54.

95. Lowe, *The Welfare State in Britain*, 320.

96. Lewis, "Developing the Mixed Economy," 183-91.

97. MacGregor and Pimlott, "Action and Inaction," 9.

98. Lowe, *The Welfare State in Britain*, 325-26.

99. V. Berridge, *AIDS in the UK: The Making of Policy, 1981-1994* (Oxford, 1996), 222.

100. ACMD, *AIDS and Drug Misuse, Part One* (London, 1988).

HOWARD I. KUSHNER

The Other War on Drugs: The Pharmaceutical Industry, Evidence-Based Medicine, and Clinical Practice

Over the past decade, evidence-based medicine (EBM) has become the standard for medical practice.[1] Evidence-based practices have been established in general medicine and specialized fields; new evidence-based journals have been launched.[2] Although its roots can be found in mid-nineteenth-century medical philosophy, contemporary EBM was largely developed by the clinical epidemiology program at McMaster University in 1992.[3] According to the McMaster manifesto published in JAMA, EBM "de-emphasizes intuition, unsystematic clinical experience, and pathophysiologic rationale as suffi-cient grounds for clinical decision-making, and stresses the examination of evidence from clinical research."[4] The most frequently cited definition of EBM is reliance on the "conscientious, explicit, and judicious use of current best evidence in making decisions about the care of individual patients," based on an integration of "individual clinical expertise with the best available external clinical evidence from systematic research."[5] However, as Stefan Timmermans and Aaron Mauck recently observed, EBM "is loosely used and can refer to anything from conducting a statistical meta-analysis of accumulated research to promoting randomized clinical trials, to supporting uniform reporting styles for research, to a personal orientation toward critical self-evaluation."[6]

Initially, EBM rejected medical practices based on anecdotal and idiosyncratic physician experiences in favor of statistically significant find-ings from population-based studies. Interventions based on individual cases or small cohorts were portrayed as suspect and quaint. Instead, prac-titioners were urged to apply findings from population-based studies to their own clinical practice. Not surprisingly, this stance resulted in more

The author thanks Claire E. Sterk for her comments and suggestions.

than a little resistance and much criticism from a number of practitioners. In response, advocates of EBM increasingly have attempted to portray it as complementary to clinical experience, and there have been calls for a more integrated approach.[7]

At bottom, EBM relies on the elaborate system of publication and peer review of medical research. It requires that health-care providers keep themselves updated on new research findings, become skilled and "efficient" literature researchers/methodologists, and learn how to apply "formal rules of evidence," including statistical analysis to critically evaluate clinical literature.[8] The challenge is to find time to do so, including the interpretation and translation of the findings as presented.[9] Although practical concerns have been raised about physicians relying on electronic databases, the validity of the data that constitutes EBM has not been widely questioned.

But what if the research and its findings are flawed or, worse, purposely misleading? What if EBM has been distorted by multinational corporations that are more concerned with profits than scientific evidence? What if pharmaceutical companies have infiltrated the medical research enterprise and have hijacked the peer-review process into a vehicle for drug marketing, including medications of questionable effectiveness and safety? These are, in fact, the claims of increasing numbers of respected members of the academic medical establishment. As a result, the validity and veracity of peer-reviewed research is being challenged, which, in turn, weakens the foundation upon which EBM is built.

The Emergence of a Consensus

Internist John Abramson, author of *Overdosed America: The Broken Promise of American Medicine* (2004) is deeply troubled by this trajectory.[10] He finds that the pharmaceutical industry has inserted itself into every aspect of medical practice from medical education to basic research and clinical care. Pharmaceutical companies have enticed a number of respectable research physicians into endorsing questionable studies, and through the use of direct advertising to patients and sophisticated marketing they have endangered the integrity of the American health-care delivery system. Abramson, now a clinical professor of medicine at Harvard, asserts that not only has the industry co-opted the mechanisms of evaluation of effective treatment for widely accepted illnesses, but also it has successfully colonized the healthy population by the construction of an array of new illnesses. This has been accomplished through the transformation of riskfactors into diseases that putatively require long-term and expensive prophylactic medications.

Like Abramson, Marcia Angell, former editor in chief of the *New England Journal of Medicine* (NEJM), now professor of social medicine at Harvard, links the near collapse of health care in the United States directly to the rise of pharmaceutical industry influence.[11] She claims this has been largely achieved through corrupting practices. For instance, Angell notes that the price of prescription drugs continues to rise, while employer insurance coverage continues to diminish. Drug companies justify their pricing policies as driven by the expense of research and development (R&D). But, according to Angell, R&D accounts form "a relatively small part of the budgets of the big drug companies—dwarfed by their vast expenditures for marketing and administration." In any case, writes Angell, the "industry is not especially innovative." They have produced very few new drugs in recent years, and those that were produced were done so through National Institutes of Health (NIH)-funded research at university medical centers, small biotech companies, and at the NIH itself. "The great majority of 'new' drugs," she writes, "are not new at all but merely variations of older drugs already on the market" but whose patents are about expire. Simply by changing one molecule, a drug company can gain a twenty-year patent and then aggressively market the slightly altered and more expensive, but not necessarily more efficacious, substance. Claims of effectiveness of these "me too" drugs are based on clinical trials that compare their actions to placebos rather than to the cheaper off-patent medications. The industry resists price regulation by wrapping itself in the flag of free enterprise while simultaneously feeding "on the unparalleled research output of American universities and the NIH. "In other words," claims Angell, "it's not private enterprise that draws them here, but the very opposite—our publicly sponsored research enterprise." Like Abramson, for Angell the pharmaceutical industry has become "primarily a marketing machine to sell drugs of dubious benefit" while using "its wealth and power to co-opt every institution that might stand in its way, including the U.S. Congress, the Food and Drug Administration, academic medical centers, and the medical profession itself."[12]

Another recent book, with the self-explanatory title, *Selling Sickness: How the World's Biggest Pharmaceutical Companies Are Turning Us All into Patients* (2005), reinforces and supplements Angell's and Abramson's analysis.[13] The co-authors, Ray Moynihan, visiting editor at the *British Medical Journal* (BMJ), and Alan Cassels, a pharmacology researcher at the University of Victoria in British Columbia, argue that "no longer content selling medicines only to the ill" the pharmaceutical industry has decided that "there's lots of money to be made telling healthy people they are sick." As a result, these firms have embarked on "slick 'awareness-raising' campaigns" aimed at "turning the worried well into the worried sick. Mild problems are painted as serious disease" and risk factors are portrayed as serious illnesses in need of pharmacological interventions.[14] For Moynihan and Cassels, "The unhealthy influence of the pharmaceutical industry has become a global scandal" that is "fundamentally distorting medical science, corrupting the way medicine is practiced, and corroding the public's trust in their doctors."[15] Unfavorable research results are eliminated from or camouflaged within the texts of industry-influenced studies. Data often are remolded in ways that present favorable results when a more transparent analysis might reveal substantial risk for patients taking the "hyped" medications.

The fear that the pharmaceutical industry has a corrosive effect on medical research and practice was reinforced in a "special communication" published in January 2006 in *JAMA* by a consortium of distinguished researchers, practitioners, and ethicists from eight of America's leading medical schools. Led by Troyen A. Brennan at Harvard and David J. Rothman at Columbia, the group warned that "the current influence of market incentives in the United States is posing extraordinary challenges to the principles of medical professionalism." They urged adoption of a series of measures aimed at insulating practitioners and academic medical researchers from potential conflicts of interests that "emanate from relationships between physicians and pharmaceutical companies and medical device manufacturers." Brennan and colleagues propose the elimination of all gifts, including pharmaceutical samples. They demanded the exclusion of physicians with financial ties to pharmaceutical companies from participating in committees that oversee purchases of medical devices, exclusion of drug companies from continuing medical education (CME) activities, and the end of direct payments for travel to meetings. Physicians were urged to cease participation in industry speakers' bureaus and to eschew the practice of authorship of ghost-written publications.[16] These recommendations reveal the growing anxiety, at least among some highly regarded and influential medical faculty, that the pharmaceutical industry has crossed a line that has placed the practice of medicine, including EBM, at dire risk.

"Taking drugs can hurt you," writes Jerry Avorn in *Powerful Medicines: The Benefits, Risks, and Costs of Prescription Drugs* (2004), and "not taking drugs can hurt you." Chief of Pharmacoepidemioloy and harmacoeconomics at Boston's Brigham and Women's Hospital and associate professor of medicine Harvard University, Avorn focuses on the risks and benefits of prescription medications. "Tens of millions of people are alive today who would be dead without their medicines, and tens of millions more have far less life-crushing disability because of prescriptions their doctors have written." But Avorn notes that "others—though mercifully a much smaller number—have become disabled or die when a drug's risk-benefit balance goes horribly wrong."[17] Like the other authors discussed in this essay, Avorn worries about the rising cost of pharmaceuticals and their impact on an already weakened medical infrastructure. For Avorn, "Every drug is a triangle with three faces, representing the healing it can bring, the hazards it can inflict, and the economic impact of each" (17). The task is to know the difference. Avorn believes that EBM, free from industry influence, provides the best vehicle for acquiring that knowledge.

Although all of these authors present similar narratives, they draw slightly different lessons and offer differing solutions for repairing what all agree is a broken system. For Abramson and Moynihan and Cassels, the problems can be traced mainly to "big Pharma's" quest for profits and its ability to seduce reputable researchers into endorsing questionable regimens and procedures. Like Abramson and Moynihan and Cassels, Avorn and Angell view the pharmaceutical industry as the villains, but they both see the solutions in structural and political reform, which they believe can ultimately be guided by an untainted EBM.

In combination, these critiques make a compelling case for the elimination of the pharmaceutical industry's influence on peer-reviewed medical research and practice. These critics assume that as a result of such reforms, EBM can provide a set of objective measures for clinical practice. However, they may underestimate the extent to which EBM itself frames medical practice in ways that undercut a patient-centered evaluation and treatment. An examination of the rhetoric of these critiques reveals an unarticulated anxiety about the role of EBM itself. This emerges in the examinations of big Pharma's subversion of physician/patient collaboration. Thus, the question remains whether elimination of industry's toxic impact on peer-reviewed medical research will ipso facto restore what putatively has been lost.

Part of the reason that the issue of impact of EBM on medical practice remains unexamined may be the focus on the compelling threats posed by the pharmaceutical industry to rational patient care. However, it also is important to explore EBM from a historical perspective. The studies discussed in this essay highlight the importance of reliable patient diagnosis, prevention, and treatment. Although the old conundrum of medical practice as an art versus medicine as a science is never directly raised, it forms much of the subtext, especially of Abramson's and Avorn's arguments.

From this perspective, it may well be that even if the goals of industry disengagement from the process of peer-reviewed clinical research is achieved, clinicians may rediscover that EBM itself provides a serious challenge to the type of medical care delivery envisioned by these authors.

I begin by reviewing the evidence laid out in four recent emblematic studies—by Abramson, Avorn, Angell, and Moynihan and Cassels—about the impact of the pharmaceutical industry on medical practice. Then, I return to EBM in historical perspective. All of these authors cover similar territory, but the structure of Abramson's *Overdosed America* serves as a useful frame, allowing us to move back and forth among these four books and some recent articles. This will prepare the ground for a return to the role of EBM.

Reexamining the Evidence

Frustrated by increasing numbers of his patients who arrive armed with drug advertisements and "a firm (if not fixed idea) of the outcome they wanted," Abramson concluded that he could best "help people to achieve better health" if he uncovered "what the scientific evidence really shows and explain this to the public."[18] What he claims to have discovered was "a scandal in medical science" equivalent to recent corporate revelations. "Rigging medical studies, misrepresenting research results published in even the most influential medical journals, and withholding the findings of whole studies that don't come out in a sponsor's favor have all become the accepted norm in commercially sponsored medical research." This corruption has been largely hidden from view by a "complex web of corporate influence that includes disempowered regulatory agencies, commercially sponsored medical education, brilliant advertising, expensive public relations campaigns, and manipulation of free media coverage." All of this is exacerbated by an interlocking financial arrangement between numerous "trusted medical experts and the medical industry" that results in conflicts of interest (xiii). According to Abramson, "There has been a virtual take-over of medical knowledge in the United States, leaving doctors and patients little opportunity to know the truth about good medical care and no safe alternative but to pay up and go along." And sadly, writes Abramson, despite the "enormous costs," both the quality and delivery of health care in America has declined.

Abramson deconstructs a number of pharmaceutical company-sponsored studies published in prestigious medical journals. These studies underpinned the aggressive advertising/marketing campaigns aimed to "educate" physicians and their patients about risk reduction. Thus he examines a *NEJM* article that claimed a 19 percent reduction in stroke risk in a population that took the statin Pravachol, compared to those who had been given a placebo.[19] However, as Abramson reminds us, the percent advantage represents the *relative* risk, but what matters is the *absolute* risk. This difference between relative and absolute risk is illustrated in Moynihan and Cassels's *Selling Sickness*, where they report a presentation given by a University of British Columbia therapeutics team, James McCormack and Bob Rango. McCormack and Rango ask their audience of baby boomers if they would take a drug for five years if (1) it lowered their risk of an MI (myocardial infarction or heart attack) by thirty-three percent (2) lowered their risk one percent, from 3 to 2 percent, (3) assured that one person in a hundred who took the drug did not have an MI, but that there was no way to predict if they would be that individual. Predictably, the majority would follow the regimen for the 33 percent reduction, fewer would opt for a mere one percent risk reduction and none would participate in the third alternative.[20] However, all three choices are the same. Thirty-three percent is the relative risk of lowering the chance of an MI from 3 to 2 percent (the absolute risk), which translates into the statistical result that 100 persons would have to take the medication for five years for one person to avoid an MI.

A close reading of the Pravachol study reveals that for every 1,000 patients who take this statin for one year there will be one less stroke. Over the six years of the clinical trial, the absolute risk advantage of taking Pravachol is a mere .8 percent. Determining the absolute risk is crucial because pharmaceutical companies advertise the putative effectiveness of a drug by its relative risk, which, as in this case, is entirely (and purposely) misleading because the typical potential drug taker at whom advertisements are aimed will assume that if they took Pravachol they would greatly reduce their chance of stroke. By emphasizing relative rather than absolute risk, drug marketing manipulates the unsophisticated statistical skills of its audience.

For Abramson, the issue of relative risk is only the beginning of the problems illustrated in the Pravachol study. For each stroke prevented (based on the price of the dose used in the study), the cost was $1.2 million—without counting the expense of blood tests, physicians visits, and patient time. But, as Abramson reveals, the study had a much more substantial flaw. The chance of a stroke increases dramatically with age and if those at greatest risk for stroke (70 and older) are separated from the general population of the study, "patients in the study age 70 and older who had been treated with Pravachol actually had 21 percent *more* strokes than patients given the placebo." Given the fact that there are a number of proven, less expensive, and less hazardous interventions that reduce stroke risk, including eating fish once a week, moderate exercise, and low-ering elevated blood pressure, the aim of the Pravachol study "seemed incontrovertible: to establish "scientific evidence," legitimated by the prestige of the *NEJM*, that would lead doctors to believe that they were reducing their patients' risk of stroke by prescribing Pravachol." In reality, asserts Abramson, the drug company was actually harming patients' health by diverting "doctors' and patients' attention away from far more effective ways to prevent stroke" (17).

The claim that stroke risk can be reduced by regular statin use has persisted, despite evidence to the contrary. Yet, as Abramson points out, a careful analysis of a 2001 *JAMA* article making that claim reveals that the lower "the total and LDL (bad) cholesterol, the *greater* the risk of stroke" (19, italics in original).[21] Although statins do raise HDL choles-terol, the level of which is important in stroke risk prevention, they were found to "raise HDL cholesterol only half as much as the article found would be necessary to significantly reduce the risk of stroke." However, "Statins lower total and LDL cholesterol at least three times more on a percentage basis, far more than enough to significantly *increase* the risk of stroke according to the data from the study" (20, italics in original).

Touted as superior in performance and safety to nonsteroidal anti-inflammatory drugs (NSAIDS), the aggressively marketed Vioxx and Celebrex ultimately proved to result in much greater incidence of serious gastrointestinal bleeding and stomach and intestinal perforation, the outcomes their manufactures promised they would reduce. The much-heralded promise of these drugs was that they would selectively inhibit pain-causing cyclooxygenase-2 (COX-2 inhibitors), but not, as with NSAIDS, also inhibit COX-1 (which protects the stomach from irrita-tion). Again, the study on which the Vioxx claim was based was published in a highly authoritative journal, the *NEJM*,[22] but as Abramson shows, a close reading of the Vioxx Gastrointestinal Outcomes Research, the so-called VIGOR clinical trial, reveals that "people who took Vioxx had twice as many heart attacks, strokes, and cardiovascular deaths and four times as many heart attacks as people who took (the NSAID) naproxen" (26). The authors of the study attempted to explain this outcome as "the play of chance," which is a very odd way to characterize a statistically significant finding, the very thing that a clinical trial is designed to uncover. The authors, two of whom had financial ties to the manufacturers of Vioxx and Celebrex, reported their finding with adjectives intended to downplay the fact that those who took these medications had increased their risk of developing heart disease and stroke more than they reduced their risk of gastrointestinal complications. As Abramson dug deeper into the research, he uncovered a web of deception and half-truths that when carefully analyzed reveal that the COX-2 inhibitors actually posed not only an unacceptable risk of heart disease and stroke to their users, but also resulted in a much greater risk of serious gastrointestinal complications than NSAIDS. Despite their own evidence that Vioxx significantly increased the risk of death for patients with prior cardiovascular disease and that Celebrex increased the risk of gastrointestinal complications, rather than reducing them, their manufacturers (Merck and Pfizer) misleadingly marketed them as safe and effective. "By the end of 2001," writes Abramson, "57 percent of all the money spent on prescription arthritis medication in the United States was spent on Celebrex and Vioxx, and both were among the top 10 selling drugs in the United States."[23]

Although the United States spends more per capita for health care than the twenty-two other OECD (Organization of Economic Cooperation and Development) industrialized nations, it is lowest in healthy life expectancy. Moreover, the United States ranks twenty-forth out of thirty-nine developed nations in terms of infant mortality. Abramson ties these statistics to the commercialization of American medicine, which has resulted in doctors prescribing "unnecessary drugs" and ordering "expensive and ineffective procedures" (53). Included in these procedures are high-dose chemotherapies followed by bone marrow transplantations like that described by Abramson of a breast cancer patient whose cancer had metastasized throughout her body. These aggressive therapies expose already sick patients to an array of additional risks, illnesses, and severe discomforts with, as in this case, no scientific evidence of efficacy. In fact, the basis for these costly interventions often is justified by shoddy or misleading studies, albeit, published in respected medical journals, often, as in this case, later proven to be based on fraudulent data (52). "I had been trained," writes Abramson, "to believe that carefully reading the medical journals, following experts' recommendations, and keeping up with continuing medical education would ensure that I was bringing the best possible care to my patients." But the opposite was so: his attempt to apply EBM "was actually subverting the quality of [his] medical care" (53).

Perhaps the most graphic example of this result is the now-well-known history of hormone replacement therapy (HRT). The basic story is told in three of these books: Abramson, Avorn, and Moynihan and Cassels. Based on faulty data and the insupportable notion that menopause was a disease rather than a natural process, millions of American women took estrogen despite evidence published in the NEJM in 1975 that estrogen replacement dramatically increased the risk of uterine cancer. Adding progestin, which putatively prevented changes in the uterine lining, and an aggressive marketing campaign to persuade women that the new combination drug, Premarin, would protect against osteoporosis and heart disease, sales skyrocketed. By the early 1990s, one out of five post-menopausal women was taking these hormones. None of these claims, however, were based on the gold-standard randomized clinical trials (RCT), until the 1998 HERS study, which revealed that rather than being protective, Premarin increased the risk of heart disease by 50 percent for women who took the drug for only one year. In fact, HRT increased the general risk of premature death. By 2005 it was clear that HRT signifi-cantly increased the risks of breast cancer, stroke, heart attacks, and blood clots. HRT led to a 15 percent increase in adverse effects for women on the regimen. "This translated into about one adverse event for every 100 women who took hormones for five years."[24] Rather than reducing the risk of Alzheimer's disease, HRT doubled it; it increased the chances of breast cancer for women taking it by 66 percent![25]

If for Abramson the HRT story challenges the efficacy of EBM, for Avorn it demonstrates its value. "How," Avorn asks, "did clinical practice lurch forward for so long and so far in the absence of solid evidence about what these products did?"[26] After all, he reminds us, "These are not obscure side-effects caused by an arcane drug; cardiovascular disease is the single most important cause of disability and death in the industrial-ized world, and HRT products were among the most widely prescribed drugs in America for years" (34). Why did it take so long for their dangers to be exposed? The reason, according to Avorn, is that "it wasn't anyone's job to make that determination." The "National Institutes of Health had initially avoided the question for years." Avorn sees this as less the result of sex bias than the NIH's "lack of interest in more mundane applied research questions about the effects of existing medications" (34). The pharmaceutical company (Wyeth) had FDA approval to market the drugs for the "temporary management of the symptoms of menopause." Although physicians routinely prescribed the drugs for other conditions that were not FDA approved, Wyeth "found it easier and safer to ride (as well as drive) the tide of prevailing medical and public opinion" (35). The company reluctantly supported the HERS study because it was persuaded that this would result in FDA approval for Premarin to be marketed as a product to reduce the risk of heart disease. Meanwhile, the FDA did nothing because it rarely enforced restrictions of off-label drug use and, in any case, the FDA does not have the resources to conduct its own clin-ical trials. "The only real hero," according to Avorn, was "the randomized clinical trial" (35).

Commercialization of American Medicine

Abramson, Angell, and Avorn agree that the current American medical system is in deep trouble. Angell views the pharmaceutical industry as the primary culprit and, along with Avorn, believes that regulation will prove the best prescription for the ailing health-care system. Although Abramson essentially endorses Angell's arguments about the corrupting power and influence of the pharmaceutical industry, he sees the problem as more complex due to what he labels "American medicine's perfect storm." Many factors—including drug companies, government, doctors, patients, insurers—have contributed to pushing the American health-care system to the edge of the "breaking point." "In the eye of the storm," Abramson sees "a single factor: the transformation of medical knowledge from a public good, measured by its potential to improve our health, into a commodity, measured by its commercial value." This is the context, argues Abramson, in which "'scientific evidence' is produced." Thus, EBM is part of the problem, rather than the solution, because in the service of commercialization "the quality of the medical information that well-informed, dedicated doctors rely on to make clinical decisions" has become corrupted (91).

The commercialization of medical knowledge has deep historical roots and can be traced to the shift in funding sources for medical research from the federal government to the private sector beginning in the 1980s. Until the 1980s, almost all support for academic medical research came from the NIH, but by 1990 the majority of submissions for support were rejected. Meanwhile, the industry dramatically increased its financial support of university-based clinical research. By 2002, 80 percent of all clinical trials were funded by the industry and, writes Abramson, drug companies "increasingly exercised the power of their purse" (95). Meanwhile, the role of academic medicine declined as pharmaceutical companies increasingly relied on for-profit research firms that were established solely for the purpose of conducting clinical trials. By hiring consultants from university faculties, "these companies could gain access to patients for clinical research through community-based doctors, or play a larger role in research design [and] data analysis" (95). The industry regularly submitted articles on their findings for publication, often recruiting academic physicians to "edit" the papers and assume primary authorship. As a result of this shift in funding, previously reluctant academic centers now actively sought industry funding. But there were strings, including agreements not to share findings with colleagues prior to publication. Abramson quotes Drummond Rennie, deputy editor of JAMA, who warned in 1999 that even the most prestigious universities "are seduced by industry funding, and frightened that if they don't go along with these gag orders, the money will go to less rigorous institutions. It's a race to the ethical bottom" (95). By 2001, the editors of twelve of the world's premiere medical journals issued a joint statement in *JAMA* warning that this corporate takeover was compromising the objectivity of medical research: clinical research, they feared, had been transformed into "a commercial activity."[27] As the editors pointed out, the impetus for commercial sponsorship of clinical trials, driven by marketing concerns, "makes a mockery of clinical investigation and is a misuse of a powerful tool." Because "many clinical trials are performed to facilitate regulatory approval of a device or drug rather than to test a specific novel scientific hypothesis," academic collaborators are recruited less for their scientific contributions than for the stamp of approval their names provide. The editors characterize this as a "draconian" system in which investigators often "have little or no input into trial design, no access to the raw data, and limited participation in data interpretation."[28]

Abramson concurs. Commercialization hijacks the research agenda by determining what gets studied and what does not. It is not "disinterested" science, but rather a project driven by the requirements of increasing sales and profits, which, as Abramson shows through a series of examples, makes it impossible for practicing physicians to trust the medical research that appears in even the most highly regarded journals.

When new drugs and devices are developed, manufacturers often market them for a wider range of patients than they were originally intended, exposing some patients to great risk. Abramson cites the history of implantable defibrillators. The manufacturer (Guidant) supported research published in the *NEJM* that suggested that the defibrillators be implanted in all heart attack patients, whether or not they had a history of ventricular fibrillation. The article suggested that if implanted in 1,000 patients, 56 would be alive at the end of twenty months who otherwise would have died. But, the study downplayed an additional finding that for each life saved by a defibrillator, there would be one additional hospitalization for congestive heart failure among patients who received an implant. The cost for each life saved would be approximately $1.5 million, not including the hospitalization bills for those who developed congestive heart failure. More important, the *NEJM* article neglected to mention that a study published previously in *Circulation*, reported that twice as many lives would be saved if the patients exercised twice weekly for one year, while the risk of congestive heart failure would decrease by 71 percent rather than increase by 33 percent. The *NEJM* article did not mention that risk would also dramatically decrease if those with heart disease reduced or ceased smoking or made other life-style alterations.

Americans spend $25 billion annually on cholesterol-reducing drugs.[29] Yet cholesterol levels represent one risk factor, among many, for coronary heart disease (CHD). A combination of aggressive marketing, abetted by researchers' conflicts of interest, has transformed a risk factor into a disease, hypercholesterolemia. Along the way, critical analysis of conflicting data has been sacrificed for enormous corporate profits. For instance, in May 2001 JAMA published an eleven-page "Executive Summary" of National Cholesterol Education Program (NCEP), guidelines on cholesterol-lowering statins. Building on the two earlier NCEP guidelines, the summary recommended "more intensive" lowering of the level of LDL cholesterol "in clinical practice." The full report is 284 pages long, and readers of the "Executive Summary" were assured that the full document was an "evidence-based and extensively referenced report that provides the scientific rationale for the recommendations contained in the executive summary."[30] However, Abramson finds that "careful scrutiny" of the full report "reveals" that "rather than presenting a balanced interpretation of the scientific findings, the report seems intent upon building the case for greater use of statins . . . and even misrepresenting findings reported in the original articles" from which the data came. Thus, Abramson concludes, "rather than promoting a balanced approach to coronary heart disease prevention and overall health promotion, the guidelines seem more intent on getting doctors to focus on lowering LDL cholesterol" (131). But, Abramson argues, lowering cholesterol "plays a relatively limited role in our overall health" (135).

What randomized clinical trials reveal, according to Abramson, is that statins may be helpful as secondary prevention for those with CHD. But the data also show no significant benefit from statins for elderly patients without heart disease. "The ultimate impact of the 2001 cholesterol guidelines," writes Abramson, "is to mislead physicians and patients." There are "inexpensive, easily accessible, and often more effective interventions [exercise, diet, and smoking cessation] to prevent heart disease and improve overall health" that "are being abandoned in favor of expensive drugs" (147).

Abramson's views are seconded by Moynihan and Cassels, who also see marketing and profits, rather than robust science, driving the use of cholesterol-reducing drugs.[31] Like Abramson, they find financial relationships between many whose publications present unambiguous endorsements of the benefits of statins. Moynihan and Cassels are troubled by the extensive list of experts who have direct ties to the pharmaceutical companies that produce these drugs. "The existence of these ties," they write, "should not imply that any of these guideline writers would make recommendations in order to please their drug company sponsors," but "the growing perception of coziness" cannot be ignored. Thus, "the doctors writing the very definitions of what constitutes high cholesterol, and recommending when drugs should be used to treat it, are at the same time paid to speak by the companies making those drugs."[32] Noting that the level of acceptable LDLs continues to be lowered, Angell writes, "I am not arguing that cholesterol levels *shouldn't* be lowered, only that this market is easily expanded and therefore rich territory for me-too drugs."[33]

Moynihan and Cassels find no evidence that statins prevent early death for healthy men and women: "For otherwise healthy people at low risk long-term use of statins may offer little benefit and unknown harms."[34] Even when appropriate, statins, according to Moynihan and Cassels, are less effective in preventing CHD than behavioral and dietary changes. They endorse Dr. Lisa Schwartz's concern that her patients believe the goal is simply to lower their cholesterol numbers, but she reminds us, what should be of concern is "whether you have lowered your risk of heart disease. Because cholesterol has become a condition, you can define a treatment's success as having a lower cholesterol level," but "the *problem* here is finding effective ways to reduce heart disease, stroke, and premature death, not cholesterol levels."[35] What the evidence indicates is that for those who do not have heart disease, statins provide only a small and not clinically significant benefit. "There is no definitive proof," conclude Moynihan and Cassels, that statins "can meaningfully contribute to the prevention of an early death" in healthy people.[36]

The authors discussed in this essay are troubled by mass marketing of pharmaceuticals to consumers. Abramson is concerned about the way drug companies use the pretense of consumer education to market drugs to a naive population, and in the process undercut the physician-patient relationship. This "hype creates false hope that moves us further away from real prevention, most of which has to do with a healthy lifestyle, and drains resources needlessly from far more effective health interventions."[37] Moynihan and Cassels believe that "one of the key ways of making healthy people believe they are sick is direct-to-consumer advertising of drugs and diseases—and there is now more than $3 billion dollars' worth of it every year in the U.S. alone," or approximately $10 million every day.[38]

Avorn is equally worried about the impact of physician-targeted educational material. "Most of us who practice medicine," writes Avorn, "are surrounded by an almost suffocating plethora of information of very uneven quality."[39] Unfortunately, information of inferior scientific value often has the greatest influence on practicing physicians. He compares medical journal articles that "are necessarily in the arid format required for rigorous scientific communication" with the materials produced by the pharmaceutical industry. "The latter are bright, colorful, engaging, with large headlines, appealing pictures, easy-to-understand graphs, and unmistakable take-home messages exhorting us to prescribe that product." Does this "ubiquitous and hardy promotional material . . . really influence how we physicians actually prescribe drugs?" he asks. "Of course it does."[40] "No one should rely on a business for impartial evaluation of the product it sells," writes Angell. "Yet the pharmaceutical industry contends it educates the medical profession and the public about its drugs and the conditions they treat, and many doctors and medical institutions—all recipients of the industry's largesse—pretend to believe it."[41] And, Angell points out, such a system distorts medical research by focusing on drugs that can return huge profits while simultaneously constraining critical analysis of effectiveness and cheaper alternative behavioral interventions. "It is easy to understand," writes Abramson, "why those profiting from this monumentally lucrative system want us to believe that market-driven health care is the best of all possible health care worlds. It is much harder to understand why doctors who have been trained to base their decisions on the best available evidence go along so willingly."[42]

Solutions

For Avorn, "The vision of medicine as just another business has made it difficult for the United States to provide the universal drug coverage" offered in all other industrialized nations.[43] Part of the solution would be "for the government to ensure that every American has coverage enough to buy a respectable health insurance package" (412). By constructing a system whose goals would be "dominated by those whose main interest is in providing appropriate medical care" (415), it would be structured to "compete on the basis of quality," where "profit-based incentives would be forbidden by law" and where the worst excesses of the current system "could be contained by aggressive legislation" (413). As a result, "hot-money of investors eager for quick profits would flee for-profit HMOs and insurers as the industry came to look more like a well-regulated public utility" (415). Avorn's plan seems to be similar to the health insurance scheme recently adopted in his home state of Massachusetts.[44]

For Abramson, the destruction of patient-based medicine by the pharmaceutical industry has been abetted by a medical education that emphasizes reduction of illness to the molecular level rather than in the context of a particular patient's wider needs. The problem can be traced, in part, to "the training and culture of medicine," which leaves "many doctors" believing that behavioral and environmental interventions "are not worthy of their skills or time." The Institute of Medicine reports that "behavior and environment are responsible for over 70 percent of avoidable mortality." The same study finds that between 10 percent and 15 percent of deaths result from inadequate medical care. Yet, 95 percent of health-care spending targets biomedical interventions, especially pharmaceuticals. "If one of the goals of medical care is to prevent disease," asks Abramson, "then, don't doctors have a professional responsibility to address the unique health needs, habits, and risks of each individual patient?"[45]

"The most important health care issue," according to Abramson, is to restore the goal of medical knowledge creation to improve the health of Americans (249). This requires four "fundamental" reforms: (1) "accurate and transparent" health information; (2) restoration of the balance of medical practitioners between primary care and specialties; (3) a health-care system that rewards providers for improving the health of patients; and (4) active government oversight to ensure that "the public's interest is being served" (256).

Angell believes that the pharmaceutical industry poses the greatest obstacle to trustworthy EBM. Therefore, her primary goal is to loosen "the iron lock of big Pharma on public policy and the medical profession"[46] This will require a series of reforms that restructure the way the industry does business. Foremost would be a shift from emphasis on "me-too" drugs to truly innovative compounds. An important step in this direction would be an FDA requirement that new substances must be compared with older drugs that treat the same conditions rather than with placebos alone. This would require a truly independent and strengthened FDA. Angell would create "an Institute for Prescription Drug Trials" within the NIH to administer prescription drug trials to ensure that "clinical trials serve a genuine medical need and that they are properly designed, conducted, and reported" (244). Angell also wants to prohibit direct-consumer advertising. Unlike other businesses, pharmaceutical companies depend on government-funded research, prolonged periods of market monopolies, and tax breaks. Because of these advantages and because of "the importance of its products to public health," the industry's financial books, disclosing the amounts spent on marketing and R&D, should be open for public scrutiny (253). Such reforms would inevitably have the effect of lowering drug prices, which, in any case, should be regulated. Finally, Angell wants to repeal the new Medicare prescription drug plan and replace it with "a simple measure that guarantees all Medicare beneficiaries appropriate coverage of their drug costs, with government-negotiated payments to industry and medically based formulary" (257).

"The obvious problem for all of us right now," write Moynihan and Cassels, "is finding good sources of information about human illness that are truly independent of drug company influence."[47] In agreement with the other authors discussed here, Moynihan and Cassels are adamant that the only way to restore trust in EBM is to insulate it from the influence of the pharmaceutical industry: to guarantee the objectivity of evidence and claims of efficacy, research must be conducted "by organizations and individuals who don't profit from selling those treatments" (198). Although their suggestions for reform are less elaborate than those offered by Abramson, Avorn, and Angell, Moynihan and Cassels are no less relentless in demanding a complete separation between big Pharma and EBM. Assuming such a detachment is possible, will EBM enable the sort of patient/physician collaboration that Abramson and Avorn hope to restore?

Patient Narratives and EBM: Medical Art Versus Science

Patient narratives pepper both Abramson's and Avorn's texts, serving to contrast the impersonal and mechanical trends and pressures placed on clinical practice with a patient-centered approach enabled by a physician's familiarity with a patient's life history. This local knowledge allows the practitioner to tailor contextualized diagnoses, treatments, and advice that mesh with individual needs. For Abramson, these case histories are exemplars of what has been lost by the triumph of a greedy pharmaceutical industry. For Avorn, patient narratives mirror the best of medical education, in which individual case studies are interrogated and, in the process, reveal why some patients fared well and others poorly when placed on similar drug regimens. These narratives are also literary devices that at once reveal Abramson's and Avorn's diagnostic and interpersonal skills, while exposing the danger of a mechanistic application of population studies. What is at stake, these stories suggest, is nothing less than the health of the very patients that EBM and the pharmaceutical industry claim to ensure. What also seems at stake, though not explicitly stated, is the survival of the art of medical practice. From this perspective, EBM itself may pose as great a challenge to the survival of the art of medicine as does the pharmaceutical industry.

As previously noted, Avorn contrasts the dry statistical presentation of medical journals with the flashy and accessible literature produced by the pharmaceutical industry. In its place, Avorn and Abramson, and to a lesser extent, Moynihan and Cassels and Angell call on patient narratives as counter-evidence for their claims. Of course, they do much more than this; but it is the clinical encounters described by Avorn and Abramson that serve as their alternative models to a therapeutics framed by evidence gleaned from population studies. From this perspective, the data gleaned from population studies and clinical trials are portrayed as a form of Galenic scholasticism, in which the skills associated with close readings of texts are characterized as of greater clinical value than the actual patient/physician encounter. The bottom line, though never fully expressed, is a call for the restoration of the clinical arts in face of an assault by an impersonal science.

"There is one aspect of medicine that will surely survive," writes Avorn, "the need for a compassionate, competent person to help another confront the suffering of illness."[48] But, as Avorn laments, it is this "oldest aspect of medicine" that "has been most fragile in our recent upheavals" (410). Despite Avorn's hope that the doctor/patient interaction "may prove the most durable in the face of the changes that are coming" (410), the evidence that he and the other authors present does not support great optimism for such an outcome. For EBM, shorn of industry influence, nevertheless presents a fundamental challenge to the idealized patient/physician interactions that Avorn and Abramson wish to restore. Although the pharmaceutical industry has served to undermine this interaction, EBM may provide, as Abramson seems to acknowledge, a greater obstacle than Avorn admits. The reasons for this are both structural and historical.

The disease mysteries and insights of the medical detectives that once populated medical journals have been relegated to the back pages. The patient increasingly has been replaced by the statistic. To the extent that patient narratives have become suspect, the insights that such cases may offer have become devalued as merely anecdotal. Moreover, human subject protection and ethics require that published cases must be sufficiently altered so that the identity of a patient will not be revealed. Thus, published patient narratives, including those provided by Avorn and Abramson, are, of necessity, "fictions." Such narratives now provide material for books, op-ed columns, films, and television programming, but not for EBM.

First and foremost, population studies underlie most of EBM. There are many reasons for this—none less compelling than the desire of contemporary medicine to be viewed as a "science" rather than an art. Dependent as it is on external funding, EBM has been enthusiastically supported by medical school administrators who judge and reward faculty by the number and dollar amount of their external grant funding. And until it became a source of controversy, EBM gained much impetus from pharmaceutical financial funding of clinical trials.

EBM requires a division of labor in which the scientific evidence is generated by researchers at prestigious research and medical institutions, while its implementation putatively takes place in the offices and clinics of practitioners. Such a system, whether intended or not, has created a growing schism between academic medicine and clinical practitioners.[49] This trend has its roots in the 1970s, when academic medicine began to distinguish itself from ordinary clinical practice by emphasizing its commitment to "research." By the 1980s, it became clear that medical "research" in itself was often problematic and not easily translated into practice. Thus, research-based medicine was augmented by the establishment of professional clinical practice guidelines based on evidence gleaned from retrospective reviews of published randomized clinical trials. "Clinical practice guidelines," writes Timmermans, were seen as a way to "capture a profession's consensus on its area of expertise and suggest the preferred way to perform an intervention."[50] It soon became apparent that physicians did not apply the guidelines consistently, if at all. "Individual autonomy," Timmermans notes, took "precedence over the prescriptive aspect of the guidelines."[51] Part of the impetus for EBM was in reaction to this continued individual autonomy and thus idiosyncratic practice. EBM provided a mechanism to ensure that academic medicine would finally trump what it viewed as the unscientific nature of medical practice. If clinical medicine were to become a "science," practice had to be based on evidence that could be replicated through testing and shown to be statistically significant. But, as Medical Historian William Rothstein reminds us, "Statistical tests are designed . . . so that very large samples make trivial differences statistically significant."[52]

Moreover, for EBM to do its work, specificity is required; each piece of data must be (as much as possible) identical to another. That is, the interpretation of an individual patient's complaints must be evaluated in deference to the findings of population studies. Art must give way to science.

In contrast, Avorn argues—beginning with the first chapter of his book—that differences among patients with similar signs and symptoms, even with the same diagnosis, can make such an application dangerous. The thrust of Abramson's initial lament is the deterioration of physician/patient collaboration. From these perspectives, it is difficult to imagine that EBM, even if liberated from the influences of the pharmaceutical industry, can provide a solution to the issues that Avorn and Abramson have identified. Despite its history of abuse, EBM continues to serve as the unquestioned standard for medical practice because it has been wrapped in the clothing of scientific objectivity and tied to the gold standard of the randomized clinical trial.

But, like all medical systems that have preceded it, EBM's triumph is rooted as much in the history as it is in science.[53] If the physician/patient collaboration that Avorn and Abramson describe is to be "restored," the knowledge claims of EBM will have to be examined with the same intensity that these authors have adopted toward the pharmaceutical industry's influence on EBM. This will require attention to both the scientific claims of EBM *and* to its historical origins.

Rollins School of Public Health
Emory University

Notes

1. Ross E. G. Upshur, "Looking for Rules in a World of Exceptions: Reflections on Evidence-Based Practice," *Perspectives in Biology and Medicine* 48 (2005): 477–89.

2. Frank Davidoff, Brian Haynes, Dave Sackett, and Richard Smith, "Evidence-Based Medicine: A New Journal to Help Doctors Identify the Information They Need," *BMJ* 310 (1995): 1085–86; David Grahame-Smith, "Evidence-Based Medicine: Socratic Dissent," *BMJ* 310 (1995): 1126–27.

3. Evidence-Based Medicine Working Group (hereafter EBMWG), "Evidence-Based Medicine: A New Approach to Teaching the Practice of Medicine," *JAMA* 268 (4 November 1992): 2420–2425.

4. Ibid., 2420.

5. David L. Sackett et al., "Evidence-Based Medicine: What It Is and What It Isn't," *BMJ* 312 (1996): 71–72.

6. Stefan Timmermans and Aaron Mauck, "The Promise and Pitfalls of Evidence-Based Medicine," *Health Affairs* 24 (2005): 18–28; 18.

7. David M. Eddy, "Evidence-Based Medicine: A Unified Approach," *Health Affairs* 24 (2005): 9–17.

8. EBMWG, "Evidence-Based Medicine," 2421–22.

9. Gordon H. Guyatt, Maureen O. Meade, Roman Z. Jaeschke, Deborah J. Cook, and R. Brian Haynes, "Practitioners of Evidence Based Care: Not All Clinicians Need to Appraise Evidence from Scratch But All Need Some Skills," *BMJ* 320 (2000): 954–55; Upshur, "Looking for Rules in a World of Exceptions," 477–89.

10. John Abramson, *Overdosed America: The Broken Promise of American Medicine* (New York, 2004).

11. Marcia Angell, *The Truth About the Drug Companies: How They Deceive Us and What to Do About It* (New York, 2004).

12. Ibid., xv–xviii. See also Marcia Angell, "Your Dangerous Drugstore," *New York Review of Books* 53(10) (2006): 38–40.

13. Ray Moynihan and Alan Cassels, *Selling Sickness: How the World's Biggest Pharmaceutical Companies Are Turning Us All into Patients* (New York, 2005).

14. Ibid., x.

15. Ibid., xii–xiii.

16. Troyen A. Brennan, David J. Rothman, and L. Blank et al., "Health Industry Practices That Create Conflicts of Interest: A Policy Proposal for Academic Medical Centers" [special communication], JAMA 25 295(4) (January 2006): 429-33.

17. Jerry Avorn, *Powerful Medicines: The Benefits, Risks, and Costs of Prescription Drugs* (New York, 2004), quotation, 17.

18. Abramson, *Overdosed America*, xii.

19. Harvey D. White, R. John Simes, Neil E. H. Anderson, and Graeme J. Hankey et al., "Pravastatin Therapy and the Risk of Stroke," *NEJM* 343 (2000): 317-26.

20. Moynihan and Cassels, *Selling Sickness*, 84-85.

21. Ralph L. Sacco, Richard T. Benson, Douglas E. Kargman, Bernadette Boden-Albala, and Catherine Tuck et al., "High Density Lipoprotein Cholesterol and Ischemic Stroke in the Elderly: The Northern Manhattan Stroke Study," *JAMA* 285, no. 21 (6 June 2001): 2729-35.

22. Garret A. FitzGerald and Carlo Patrono, "The Coxibs, Selective Inhibitors of Cyclooxygenase-2," *NEJM* 345, no. 6 (9 August 2001): 433-42.

23. Angell has recently endorsed and updated Abramson's arguments. Angell, "Your Dangerous Drugstore," 38-40.

24. Abramson, *Overdosed America*, 68.

25. A recent re-analysis review of the HERS data has led some researchers to conclude that for most women HRT is safe. "Based on available data, the benefits of hormone therapy outweigh the risks," according to Phillips and Langer. "Most women should receive hormone therapy at menopause." They suggest that "those women who start taking estrogen at menopause and do well should continue on hormone therapy, but it may be wise to change from MPA to progesterone. Starting hormone therapy late after menopause may be considered for women with major osteoporosis that is not responsive to other treatments." Lawrence S. Phillips and Robert D. Langer, "Postmenopausal Hormone Therapy: Critical Reappraisal and a Unified Hypothesis," *Obstetrical & Gynecological Survey* 60, no. 8 (2005): 525-26.

26. Avorn, *Powerful Medicines*, 34.

27. Frank Davidoff, Catherine D. DeAngelis, Jeffrey M. Drazen, John Hoey, and Liselotte Hojgaard et al., "Sponsorship, Authorship, and Accountability" [editorial], JAMA 286, no. 10 (12 September 2001): 1232-34.

28. Ibid., 1232-33.

29. Moynihan and Cassels, *Selling Sickness*, 1-3.

30. Expert Panel on Detection, Evaluation, and Treatment of High Blood Cholesterol in Adults, "Executive Summary of the Third Report of the National Cholesterol Education Program (NCEP) Expert Panel on Detection, Evaluation, and Treatment of High Blood Cholesterol in Adults (Adult Treatment Panel III)"[special communication], JAMA 285 (16 May 2001): 2486-97, quotations p. 2486.

31. Moynihan and Cassels, *Selling Sickness*, 1-3.

32. Ibid., 4.

33. Angel, *The Truth About the Drug Companies*, 85-86 (italics in original).

34. Moynihan and Cassels, *Selling Sickness*, 11.

35. Ibid., 12-13 (italics in original).

36. Ibid., 14.

37. Abramson, *Overdosed America*, 166.

38. Moynihan and Cassels, *Selling Sickness*, 12.

39. Avorn, *Powerful Medicines*, 293.

40. Ibid.

41. Angell, *The Truth About the Drug Companies*, 135.

42. Abramson, *Overdosed America*, 185.

43. Avorn, *Powerful Medicines*, 411.

44. Pam Belluck, "Massachusetts Sets Health Plan for Nearly All," *New York Times*, 5 April 2006, A1; David A. Fahrenthold, "Mass. Bill Requires Health Coverage State Set to Use Auto Insurance as a Model," *Washington Post*, 5 April 2006, A01.

45. Abramson, *Overdosed America*, 204-5.

46. Angell, *The Truth About the Drug Companies*, 240.

47. Moynihan and Cassels, *Selling Sickness*, 197.

48. Avorn, *Powerful Medicines*, 410.

49. Eddy, "Evidence-Based Medicine: A Unified Approach," 16; Timmermans and Mauck, "The Promise and Pitfalls of Evidence-Based Medicine," 21.

50. Timmermans, "From Autonomy to Accountability," 494.

51. Ibid.

52. William G. Rothstein, *Public Health and the Risk Factor: The History of an Uneven Medical Revolution* (Rochester, N.Y., 2003), 366.

53. For a fuller discussion of this history, see Rothstein, *Public Health and the Risk Factor*; Sidney A. Halperin, *Lesser Harms: The Morality of Risk in Medical Research* (Chicago, 2005); and Harry Marks, *The Progress of Experiment: Science and Therapeutic Reform in the United States, 1900–1990* (New York, 1997).

CONSTANCE A. NATHANSON

The Contingent Power of Experts: Public Health Policy in the United States, Britain, and France

Dangers to life and health abound. Even among the subset known to medicine and science, however, there is no guarantee that any particular danger will rise to the level of a recognized public health problem or elicit a response from the makers of public policy. The path from knowledge to policy is not straightforward; scientific consensus does not lead automatically to policy consensus. Judgments of what dangers should be most feared, how to explain them, what to do about them, and even whether they are public health problems at all are the outcome of social processes.[1] A couple of examples may help to clarify these points.

In 1865—nearly twenty years in advance of Robert Koch's better-known discoveries—Jean-Antoine Villemin reported to the French Academy of Medicine that tuberculosis was a specific disease, transmissible by inoculation between animals and from man to animals.[2] Villemin was a highly respected scientist, elected to the Academy in recognition of his work, his credentials impeccable. Nevertheless, his conclusions that tuberculosis was a contagious disease and that appropriate precautions should be taken were rejected not once but repeatedly by the Academy of Medicine.[3] His conclusions were rejected not because his colleagues doubted his science but because they found the implications of his conclusions—for their own actions, for their patients, and for the relation between doctor and patient—socially and morally unacceptable. If tuberculosis was contagious, then its victims were dangerous to their family and friends and, one physician said in a speech to the Academy of Medicine, "'What a calamity such a result would be! . . . [P]oor consumptives sequestered like lepers; the tenderness of [their] families at war with fear and selfishness.' The possibility was too

An earlier version of this paper was presented at the Workshop on Population Knowledge sponsored by the International Union for the Scientific Study of Population, Brown University, Providence, Rhode Island, 20-24 March 2001.

horrible for him to contemplate. 'If consumption is contagious, we must say so in whispers' (*Si la phthisie est contagieuse, il faut le dire tout bas*)."[4] Mandatory notification of tuberculosis cases to public health authorities did not become law in France until 1963, nearly one hundred years after Villemin had published his results.[5]

I owe my second example to the work of Karen Litfin on contemporary international efforts to regulate risks to the global environment.[6] She contrasts the *relatively* successful action to limit destruction of the ozone layer embodied in the Montreal Protocol signed in 1987 by twenty-four countries (on which her monograph primarily focuses) with the inaction of governments in response to the threat of global climate change ("greenhouse gases"). There is broad scientific consensus that climate change is a "very, very real problem" and that the "social and environmental damage from global climate change is likely to be far more catastrophic than that caused by ozone depletion."[7] There is, nevertheless, substantial scientific uncertainty as to the degree and timing of climate change; the costs of regulation are (as in my first example) perceived by policy and political actors as extremely high; the benefits (as well as costs) of action are unevenly distributed among rich and poor countries; and—perhaps most important—the risks of inaction are, at least in the short term, largely invisible. Immediate and credible threats (real or manufactured) are more often than not a *sine qua non* for public health action.[8] The effects of climate change have not so far offered opportunities for the portrayal of risks comparable to the rhetorically and visually dramatic Arctic "ozone hole." And so, despite a strong scientific consensus in favor of regulatory action, opponents of action have so far prevailed.[9]

Policymakers require authoritative advice. Authority in public health is presumed to reside with experts in medicine and public health. Nevertheless, as the forgoing examples demonstrate, the credibility of experts and their power relative to other actors in the dramas of public health are limited, subject to a variety of contingencies. In this article, I identify and examine those contingencies in some detail, based on comparative cross-national research on policymaking in public health. I conclude that expert credibility and the authority of knowledge are contingent on the characteristics of political regimes; on the social and political location as well as the framing expertise of "knowledge brokers"; and on fortuitous conjunctions of timing and opportunity.[10] My analysis of these contingencies is based on examination of public health campaigns against smoking and against HIV/AIDS in injection drug users as carried out in the United States, Britain, and France. I begin with two brief case studies that highlight the contingent role of "knowledge" in these campaigns.[11] I then develop and illustrate a series of propositions that identify the structural and normative character of these contingencies in more specific terms.

The goal of this exercise is to contribute to a more general theory of the relations between knowledge, power, and public policy.

Smoking: Environmental Pollutant or Addictive Drug?

The first, and the most important, milestones in the medical case against tobacco were laid down in the 1950s and 1960s, signaled by the publication in 1962 of the report of the Royal College of Physicians of London, *Smoking and Health,* and by the U.S. Surgeon General's report of the same name in 1964.[12] In neither report was there any reference to "passive smoking" or to the rights of the nonsmoker.[13] Smoking was construed as dangerous to the health of the smoker; the innocent bystander had yet to be discovered. References to addiction, while not absent, were muted. The Surgeon General's Report analogized smoking to coffee, tea, and cocoa—not, as in more recent reports, to heroin and cocaine. The Royal College allowed that "smokers may be addicted to nicotine," but thought that "social factors play a bigger part in determining smoking habits than internal drives or needs."[14]

Authoritative reports by recognized scientific bodies focused specifically on the hazards of "environmental tobacco smoke" (ETS) and on the addictive properties of nicotine did not, in fact, begin to appear until the mid-1980s. The relevant Surgeon General's reports were published in 1986 ("involuntary smoking") and 1988 (nicotine addiction); the National Research Council weighed in on "environmental tobacco smoke" in 1986.[15] In Britain, what came to be known as the "Froggatt report," identifying "ETS" as a danger to nonsmokers, came out in 1988.[16] A comparably authoritative report was published in France in 1997.[17] The significance of these reports did not lie in their scientific originality but in the imprimatur of scientific credibility and "official" legitimacy conferred on one side of an ongoing argument about risks. However, the relative importance of this imprimatur to the case against tobacco has been highly variable both cross-nationally and as between ETS and addiction.

Observers of the tobacco-control movement in the United States have commented on "the softness of the scientific case against second-hand smoke" prior to the 1980s, assuming that a strong scientific case was essential to the country's nonsmokers' rights movement.[18] It was not. Between 1954 and 1970, the percentage of the American public who "agreed" that cigarette smoking causes lung cancer had increased from 41 to 70 percent[19]. An authoritative case for the hazards of smoking had been made. Little more in the way of scientific evidence was required for antismoking advocates to argue that *involuntary* exposure to this deadly product was dangerous to nonsmokers. In January 1971, the then Surgeon General (Jesse L. Steinfeld) urged the adoption of a "Bill of Rights for the Nonsmoker," including a ban on smoking in "all confined public places."[20] Almost simultaneously, and of much greater significance in the long run, the nonsmokers' rights movement was launched.

The Group Against Smokers' Pollution (GASP) was founded in Maryland in early 1971.[21] From its inception, GASP's mission was twofold: first, to "get nonsmokers to protect themselves" against the immediate, irritating effects of cigarette smoke and, second, "to make smoking so unpopular that smokers would quit" (interview with GASP founder Clara Gouin, 11/4/95). In the first paragraph of the first number of its newsletter, published in March 1971, GASP called on innocent nonsmokers, the "involuntary victims of tobacco smoke," to rise up and assert their "right to breathe clean air [which] is superior to the right of the smoker to enjoy a harmful habit."[22] With the benefit of the American Lung Association's silent partnership, *The Ventilator* went out to ALA chapters throughout the country. Buttons ("GASP—non-smokers have rights, too") and posters were offered, plus a subscription to the newsletter for $1.00 a year. The response was far beyond the group's anticipation, both in the media and in recruitment to the movement for nonsmokers' rights. GASP chapters were quickly formed in Berkeley and San Francisco. By 1974, the newsletter listed fifty-six local chapters, two in Canada. The focus of nonsmokers' rights activists shifted in the mid-1970s from passing out leaflets and buttons to the passage of state and local antismoking regulations. These activities generated increased publicity, brought new groups and individuals into the movement (for example, some local chapters of the American Cancer Society), and created new demands for organization and for legal (not scientific) expertise. What began as a grassroots social movement became an organizational field.[23]

It is hard to overstate the importance for smoking behavior change in the United States of the rhetorical shift from smokers' health to nonsmokers' rights. The hazards of smoking were relocated from the individuals' risky behavior to the behavior of his smoking neighbor; risk-taking was no longer a matter of "choice" but of victimization; and, most critically, the responsibility for risk reduction was shifted away from the individual "at risk" to the "polluting" smoker and to the regulatory agencies of government. The tobacco industry recognized the power of this new construction almost immediately: "The most potentially dangerous threat to the future of the tobacco industry" a spokesperson stated in 1973, "[is] the developing psychological attitude that smoking is somehow socially unacceptable."[24] Confirming the industry's fears, a 1978 report by the Roper organization concluded that "the nonsmokers' rights movement was the single greatest threat to the viability of the tobacco industry."[25] The question of a causal relation between the nonsmokers' rights movement and the decline in cigarette consumption in the United States during the 1970s was directly addressed by Kenneth Warner in a paper published in *Science* in 1981.[26] Warner used multiple regression techniques to take account of changes in media attention to smoking's health effects and in cigarette taxation and concluded that "both declining consumption and growth in legislation [restricting smoking in public places] probably reflect a prevailing nonsmoking ethos" induced by the movement for nonsmokers' rights.[27] This paper is particularly important for the time period to which it refers, almost a decade before the publication of "authoritative" knowledge on the effects of ETS.

Nicotine addiction has had a strikingly different trajectory, particularly in the United States. The addictive properties of nicotine had "been common knowledge in medical and public health circles for years."[28] The linkage signaled by the 1988 Surgeon General's report did not reflect new scientific knowledge but rather the increased vulnerability of the tobacco industry and the shifting political and legal strategies of its opponents.[29] Among other things, the fact that "medical and public health circles" knew that nicotine was an addictive drug proved to be a far less powerful "fact" than that the tobacco industry knew it as well. The companies' knowledge was critical to litigation against them, but the discovery of their knowledge had an impact beyond mere lawyerly concerns, perhaps akin to the discovery of Oedipus' parentage in Sophocles' play.

The "addiction" label allowed antitobacco advocates in the United States to make the identical argument that had been drawn from the discovery of ETS: exposure to the dangers of smoking is not a "choice." "*The Health Consequences of Smoking: Nicotine Addiction* provided a comprehensive review of the evidence that cigarettes and other forms of tobacco are addicting and that nicotine is the drug in tobacco that causes addiction. These two factors refute the argument that smoking is a matter of free choice. Most smokers start smoking as teenagers and then become addicted."[30] This construction has a number of consequences. It was the basis for the Food and Drug Administration's (unsuccessful) efforts to regulate cigarettes as drug delivery devices; it gave plaintiffs' lawyers a counter-argument against the industry's long-standing claim that smokers "assume the risk" of their behavior; it enabled opponents to characterize tobacco industry executives as "drug dealers" and to play on deep-seated American fears of adolescent vulnerability to seduction by unscrupulous predators.

While the dangers of passive smoking and the addictive properties of cigarettes have played important roles in British and French tobacco war discourse and policymaking, the meanings attributed to these public health threats, their status as "knowledge," and the paths between knowledge and policy have been very different, both as compared with the United States and as between the two European countries. The risks of passive smoking were placed on the public agenda in Britain by an expert committee of scientists, in France by the executive branch of government acting through Parliament.[31] In neither case did nonsmokers' rights organizations play a role in these policy actions. The organizations were unimportant not because they did not exist but for other reasons: they were relatively small and weak; their adherents were discounted as "zealots"; and they lacked "scientific" authority.

Comparing the strategies of British and American antitobacco advocates, a former head of ASH (the principal antismoking advocacy group in Britain) commented wonderingly that the Americans "concentrated on passive smoking, really, well before that thing was even invented"(interview, 1998). Among the most striking contrasts between the two countries is the skittish approach of every prominent actor in Britain's tobacco wars to the question of nonsmokers' rights and, in particular, to the "energetic zealots" perceived as advocating those rights.[32] The activist role of a grassroots nonsmokers' rights movement in the United States was played in Britain by socially and/or politically well-connected physicians and organized medicine, and their focus was on industry advertising and sponsorship, not on passive smoking.[33] During the period when passive smoking was the central theme of antitobacco advocacy in the United States (the 1970s and early 1980s), there was an almost complete absence of rhetoric around this issue in Britain. It was not until 1988, following publication of the Froggatt report, in which passive smoking was accorded the legitimacy of "science," that the idea of nonsmokers as innocent victims gained credibility in Britain. Once this argument was accepted, however, its impact was as profound in Britain as it had been in the United States: "Here was a risk to the general population rather than just to the individual smoker. . . . At a stroke, this widened the debate and provided a more powerful engine for driving policy."[34]

Belief in the authority of science and distrust of energetic zealots are as much part of the public health policymaking environment in France as in Britain. French antismoking policies were shaped by medical specialists in oncology, chest diseases, and public health. However, the resemblance ends there. Smoking (passive and otherwise) has had questionable legitimacy as a public health issue in France in part because it was perceived by many physicians and scientists to be *inherently* not science but advocacy. Further, while the credibility of medically backed statements about the dangers of smoking were largely unquestioned by politicians, intellectuals, and the public, the *government's* credibility as prime translator of these statements into policy was highly suspect. So the question was not about the scientific merits of the case against *tabagisme passif* but about the balance to be struck between the liberty of the individual to smoke and the government's responsibility for protecting public health.[35]

Measures for protection of the nonsmoking public against cigarette smoke were included in France's first (1976) tobacco legislation, long before the appearance of credible scientific evidence of danger to nonsmokers and with no public or even significant parliamentary discussion.[36] These measures were not much noticed, nor were they enforced. In 1991 considerably more stringent measures were passed, again with little debate. This time, however, the reaction was powerful. The French press identified what was perceived to be a privileging of nonsmokers over smokers as the heart of this new legislation (it was not so perceived by the bill's authors). Fierce debate ensued in which the state's role in public health was alternately portrayed as one of benevolent protector or totalitarian despot. Clearly, this debate had little to do with science.

Smoking as addiction and the bundling of tobacco with marijuana, heroin, and cocaine have had a recent revival in British and French tobacco war discourse, as they have in the United States. A longtime British smoking researcher suggested in 1995 that by the 1990s the scientific paradigm of smoking had shifted from epidemiology and passive smoking to addiction.[37] In France, tobacco was recently designated as a drug within the purview of the *Mission interministerielle de lutte contre la drogue et la toxicomanie* (MILDT) along with heroin, cocaine, and marijuana. However, the significance of this shift is quite different in Britain and France from in the United States. In the United States, addiction rhetoric is used to blunt the argument that smokers knowingly court danger as a matter of choice (and as a club with which to beat the tobacco industry), while in the two European countries "addiction" is a vehicle for medicalizing—and hence depoliticizing—smoking, thus shifting the battlefield from the courts and parliament to the consulting room.

HIV/AIDS in Injection Drug Users: The Battle over Harm Reduction

Whereas sex between men is the principal mode of HIV transmission in the industrialized countries of the West, its relative magnitude has declined over time. Injection drug use was a significant mode of transmission from the beginning of the AIDS epidemic. In all three countries its importance as a percentage of reported cases peaked in the mid-1990s, but at very different levels. In 1995 more than a quarter of AIDS cases in the United States and France were attributed to injection drug use as compared with 9 percent in the UK. These percentages have since declined, but the ranking of the three countries remains the same.[38]

Recommended strategies for prevention of HIV infection among injection drug users have included abstinence from drug use, substitution of a noninjectable narcotic drug (e.g., methadone) for drug injection, needle sterilization before each use (e.g., with bleach), and arrangements to provide injection drug users with sterile equipment. "For injection drug users who cannot or will not stop injecting drugs, the once-only use of sterile needles and syringes remains the safest, most effective approach for limiting HIV transmission."[39] In industrialized countries, the two principal means advocated by public health authorities for preventing HIV infection among injection drug users are substitution and the use of sterile injection equipment.

On April 20, 1998, following considerable media buildup, the Clinton administration announced, on the one hand, that a "meticulous scientific review has now proven that needle exchange programs can reduce the transmission of HIV and save lives without losing ground in the battle against illegal drugs" and, on the other hand, that a ban on federal funds for such programs, first imposed in 1988, would remain in place. In 1997 an NIH Consensus Development Statement on the "Effective Medical Treatment of Heroin Addiction" recommended that restrictive federal methadone regulations in place since 1972 should be eliminated entirely. Addiction should be treated as a disease, and "many more physicians and pharmacies" should be allowed to prescribe and dispense methadone. It is almost needless to say that there has been no action on this recommendation.

Both the Institute of Medicine of the National Academy of Sciences and the National Institutes of Health have conducted detailed scientific reviews of needle exchange and methadone maintenance.[40] The expert committees might have saved their breath. In the United States, HIV/AIDS among injection drug users has been designated as a drug problem, not a problem in the prevention of infectious disease. The causes of this construction lie deep in the century-long history of narcotic drug-control policy in this country. Its consequences are manifold. Their end result is to seriously limit the authority of public health experts to prescribe and of the federal government to fund an effective response to HIV/AIDS in the injecting drug use population.[41]

In Britain, HIV/AIDS in injection drug users was recognized as a problem by local physicians in Edinburgh in the mid-1980s and generated its full share of expert committees. The policy response to those committees' reports was, however, very different than in the United States. The first such report was issued by the Scottish Home and Health Department in September 1986. The first sentence of the report's first recommendation was, "Injecting drug misusers who cannot or will not abstain from misuse must be educated in *safer drug taking practices*" (emphasis mine).[42] This recommendation was based on the committee's stated premise that "infection with HIV poses a much greater threat to the life of the individual than the misuse of drugs."[43] Two years later, a UK-appointed advisory group—the Advisory Committee on the Misuse of Drugs (ACMD)—reached the same conclusion: "HIV is a greater threat to public and individual health than drug misuse."[44] The committee's recommendations called for "access to sterile needles and syringes" for those who will not stop injecting and for "prescribing" as a means of "attracting drug misusers to services and helping them move away from HIV risk behaviour."[45]

The ACMD was composed of experts in medicine and public health. The British government accepted this committee's premises and acted on its recommendations. Fifteen "pilot" syringe-exchange schemes were initiated in 1987, and "syringe-exchange rapidly became the hub of HIV prevention."[46] Between 1987 and 1994 there was a fourteen-fold increase in targeted funding for this purpose; by 2002, "27 million syringes were distributed annually from over 2000 outlets in the United Kingdom."[47]

These policy initiatives emerged in a public and political opinion climate not so different from that in the United States. Serious alarm about drug "misuse" (the British term of art) in general and heroin addiction in particular surfaced in political speeches and the popular press in the early 1980s and was reflected in legislation containing substantially increased penalties for drug trafficking.[48] The major differences between the two countries were, first, the long—if recently uneven—British history of treating the use of narcotic drugs as a problem legitimately within the purview of medical experts; second, the "hermetically-sealed" British political system that allows controversial policies to be decided and implemented by "delicate manoeuvering, parliamentary persuasion and political stealth"[49]; third, the fortuitous circumstance that community-based programs for drug users had been initiated by civil servants within the British Department of Health before the advent of the AIDS epidemic. In very brief summary, the government's response to HIV/AIDS in injection drug users emerged out of "an essentially private world where policy was made by accommodation between experts and civil servants."[50] Public opinion played virtually no role, at least none acknowledged either in the many published accounts of these events nor in my interviews with key players.[51] The voices of voluntary organizations and advocacy groups, insofar as they were heard at all, were channeled through government-appointed advisory committees of "the great and the good."

In 1994, the French government authorized distribution of clean needles by nonprofit organizations and pharmacy sales of methadone on physician prescription pursuant to the recommendations of its expert committee known as the Henrion Commission. The French action came ten years after French epidemiologists had called attention to a significant problem of HIV/AIDS among injection drug users, and it lagged seven years behind similar action in Britain. The reasons for this lag are complex. It resulted from conflict among "experts" and between experts and representatives of the criminal-justice system over the meaning and treatment of narcotic drugs and narcotic drug use and also from policymakers' fear of political backlash from the Far Right.

In France, drug addiction is defined as a psychiatric problem, drug-treatment specialists are psychiatrists, and the treatment of choice is psychoanalysis. The professional ideology to which these specialists subscribe demands that treatment for drug addiction be "voluntary, anonymous, and free."[52] The patient must "want" to be cured. These principles are in conflict not only with major provisions of French drug law but also with the relative priority assigned by public health authorities (in France as elsewhere) to disease prevention as compared with the "misuse" of drugs.[53]

French law (passed in 1970) criminalizes drug *use* but provides that an individual can avoid prosecution for this offense by submitting to treatment with a view to the "cure" of his or her addiction, that is, abstinence. The drug treatment community rejected the coercive implications of this law along with the role in implementation of the law to which treatment specialists were assigned. The number of slots for psychiatric treatment remained far below the potential demand, and the law is not enforced. Hostility to what became known as the "therapeutic injunction" was equaled, if not surpassed, by hostility to "medicalization": the public health construction of drug addiction as a chronic disease requiring ongoing medical treatment. From this latter perspective—a perspective that is, perhaps, the most difficult for an outsider to understand—defining drug addiction as an organic illness had two destructive consequences. First, it was equivalent to giving up on the therapeutic goal of abstinence—"abandoning drug addicts to their addiction." Second, treatment in the form of *substitution*–insofar as the patient was both dependent on the physician and subjected to continuous monitoring for compliance with the treatment regimen–was (like the therapeutic injunction) simply another form of "social control."[54] The authorities on drug treatment in France–the authorities routinely consulted by government officials, politicians, and journalists–were firmly committed to treatment of the drug user's "soul" and firmly against treatment of the user's body. These specialists controlled the drug treatment bureaucracy to which narcotic drug users were routinely referred, a bureaucracy that preexisted, and was completely separate from, the agencies created by the French government to cope with AIDS.

A second major contributor to the delay in addressing HIV/AIDS in injection drug users was the politicization of the AIDS/drugs nexus by Jean-Marie Le Pen's ultraconservative National Front. Le Pen advocated the criminalization of homosexuality and the quarantine of AIDS victims. Health professionals and mainstream politicians of both the Left and the Right were united in their fear that to call attention to the AIDS/drugs connection was to play into Le Pen's hands. In the wake of past and prospective political gains by Le Pen and his followers in the late 1980s, these fears were an additional deterrent to open confrontation with France's AIDS epidemic.

The policy impasse was finally broken by external pressures on the government: the HIV-contaminated blood scandal that erupted in the early 1990s and caused public officials to become "very afraid of not taking extremely seriously this question of drugs"; and the sudden mobilization of a few French AIDS experts and drug-treatment workers following the eighth international AIDS conference held in Amsterdam in 1992.[55]

Among the most important obstacles to public health action in France is that public health itself is both ideologically suspect and institutionally weak. The identification of public health with social control is firmly embedded in the political culture of the French Left.[56] State regulation in the interest of disease and accident prevention (such as smoking restrictions, mandated seat-belt use, even methadone maintenance to prevent HIV infection) is characterized by intellectuals of this persuasion as deprivation by an overprotective (even quasi-totalitarian) state of individuals' right to enjoy dangerous pleasures.[57] From this perspective, only the enemies of liberty sound the public health alarm. At the same time, public health is institutionally weak both with respect to other government ministries and with respect to other sources of expertise (e.g., psychiatrists) on questions of health and illness.[58]

The Contingent Power of Experts

Authoritative knowledge is, in principle, essential to the definition and analysis of dangers to the public's health and to the deployment of an effective response. How and by whom this knowledge is framed, to whom it is addressed, and its relative acceptability have shifted with time and circumstance. The detailed case studies of smoking and AIDS/drugs not only exemplify the variability and negotiability of expert knowledge but also provide the basis for inferences about the nature of these contingencies

Regime contingencies. In comments on the difference between "hierarchical" and "individualistic" political cultures, Mary Douglas remarks that "each type of culture is based on a distinctive attitude toward knowledge."[59] In hierarchical systems (exemplified in this paper by Britain and France), the political consensus that upholds the regime itself simultaneously guarantees the authority of accredited experts and of the "knowledge" they purvey. In an individualistic system (exemplified by the United States), experts compete in the open marketplace, and their "knowledge" must be defended at every turn. Jasanoff makes much the same point with specific reference to the credibility of statements about risk: "Differences in the societal response to risk between the United States and other nations result in part from the relatively low level of scientific pluralism in countries with a more homogenous or centralized culture of knowledge."[60]

Paralleling the normative distinction between competing and consensual "cultures of knowledge" is a structural difference in the *pathways* by which expert knowledge enters the political system and becomes part of the policy decision process. Centralized ("hierarchical") regimes employ a strategy of incorporation in which the potentially competing voices of interested parties are muted by a process of channeling through the structures of government (and those voices that do not make the cut are left out). The strategy employed in decentralized ("individualistic") regimes is one of "pluralist competition" that encourages mobilization outside of government.[61]

These distinctions are of course relative and may be diminishing over time. Nevertheless, they help to account for the cross-national differences I have described in the relation of knowledge to power. In Britain the national government wields significant power in the domain of public health through its executive branch. Credible public health knowledge is monopolized and deployed by a limited number of government-appointed experts who conduct much of their business in secret. The dominant British model of science is "a craft activity involving accumulated experience and refined intuition, which cannot be formally specified, codified, and externally checked. Only other mature experts can judge, and their judgements are legitimately inaccessible except to a privileged (and socially trustworthy) few."[62] This craft activity is embodied in scientific committees of "the great and the good." The influence of these committees is exemplified by the success of the ACMD in conferring legitimacy on needle-exchange programs and by the lag in recognition of passive smoking until the Froggatt Committee had spoken. With these committees' endorsement in hand, the government acted swiftly without much regard to negative public or political opinion.[63] For better or worse, this is a regime in which debate on what are defined as health issues is dominated by medical and professional knowledge and opinion, and politicization of these issues is limited.

At almost the opposite extreme is the United States, where no single group has a scientific monopoly, where knowledge is highly contested, and where there is considerable mistrust of scientific authority. The dangers of passive smoking were promoted by locally based advocacy groups and were made the grounds for state and local regulation in places of public accommodation without the benefit of *scientific* authority beyond that of the 1964 Surgeon General's report. At the same time, no amount of authoritative pronouncements by expert committees has been able to budge the federal government's position against funding what are recognized worldwide as the most effective preventive measures against the transmission of HIV through injection drug use. What these two seemingly disparate cases have in common is the minor role played by certifiably "scientific" knowledge relative to other interests.

The *New York Times* ran an ad a few years ago from the advocacy organization *Tom Paine.com* depicting a physician with a lighted cigarette in his hand. The statement that balloons from his mouth is, "Trust us, we're experts!" The gist of the ad is that "polluters," "Big Tobacco," and "agribusiness" employ "'independent experts'–third parties who produce research and pronouncements promoting what their corporate sponsors want the public and the media to believe" (2/2001 op-ed page). The ad does not say whose experts *should* be believed, no doubt those anointed by a right-thinking (some, of course, would quip left-thinking) body like Tom Paine. It reflects (and, of course, contributes to) a reality in which there is no hierarchically based political regime to accredit one source of knowledge more than another. In such a system knowledge is politicized, and "spin" (or framing processes, to use the technical term) becomes all important, as I will discuss below.

In the framework I have described, France presents multiple paradoxes. From the perspective of virtually every historian and political scientist who has written about the country, France is the classic example of a "highly centralized and activist state."[64] Political and administrative authority are in the hands of a technocratic elite, virtually all of whom are graduates of the same set of elite educational institutions (*les grands écoles*). Indeed, notes the foremost American authority on this elite, Ezra Suleiman, "the [political] system does not make much allowance for any recognition or reward of competence that has not been certified by the elite institutions."[65] Furthermore, elite intellectual culture as well as intellectuals themselves have substantial social and political influence and prestige.[66] Their pronouncements are aired by the national media and their activities and lifestyles recorded and followed. The other side of this coin is that groups, individuals, and ideas not certified by elite institutions or public intellectuals may find themselves effectively blocked from influence on public policy. Their "knowledge" is not taken seriously and there are few alternative points of access to political decision makers. In the domain of public health, the French "highly centralized and activist state" is its own worst enemy.

The government's health and social ministries, Jobert points out, are the last choice of the weakest *grands écoles* graduates.[67] Civil servants charged with health administration have little prestige or power within the executive and are largely disdained and distrusted by the physicians for whom they have oversight responsibility. In these circumstances public health policy change is driven either by crises, as in the case of the scandal over HIV-tainted blood supplies,[68] or by activists outside the government who are themselves members of the intellectual elite or have been successful in garnering elite endorsement and support, as in the case of tobacco control and AIDS/drugs policies. It is perhaps the ultimate paradox that in a society that reveres its intellectuals, knowledge—however well grounded in medicine and science—has little chance of entering policymakers' calculations without the imprimatur of publicly recognized elites.

Belief contingencies. What qualifies as knowledge depends in part on the normative beliefs of political gatekeepers. Certifiable knowledge legitimates policy decisions, and the demand for technological and scientific knowledge to guide, inform, and frequently bolster public policy is enormous. Policymakers need experts. Yet expert analysis and advice is filtered through policymakers' political requirements and ideological beliefs.

The "knowledge" that clean needles protect against HIV transmission without increasing drug use has been replicated repeatedly and is widely diffused in the relevant scientific journals as well as in the reports of governments and international bodies. Similarly, the value of methadone as a substitute for heroin injection that both avoids the dangers of injection and allows users to lead normal and productive lives has been fully demonstrated. However, knowledge is power only insofar as the powerful allow. The accumulated knowledge of effective measures for disease prevention among injection drug users conflicted with the normative beliefs of U.S. policymakers in the immorality of drug use and the priority of the war on drugs over the prevention of disease. The same knowledge conflicted with the belief of politically influential French psychoanalysts in a particular model of drug treatment and with the concern of French policymakers about providing an opening to the politically far right wing.

"Knowledge broker" contingencies: status and expertise. Knowledge brokers are the interpreters of science. Among these brokers are, of course, scientists themselves and the scientific journalists who write about their work. Other actors may play this role as well. In addition to persons at various levels of government,

> nongovernmental actors, including social movements and business, can also function as knowledge brokers, framing and translating information not only for decision makers but also for the media and the public. Thus, while scientific knowledge is an important source of power, scientists are not the only ones with access to it; once produced, knowledge becomes something of a collective good, available to all who want to incorporate it into their discursive strategies.[69]

The relative influence of these various categories of knowledge broker depends in part on the nature of the political regime. Nongovernmental knowledge brokers have many more points of access to policy decision makers in the "pluralist" polity of the United States than in the more centralized polities of Britain and France. Influence is dependent as well, however, on knowledge brokers' local and/or national prestige (or access to prestigious support networks) and on their expertise at framing knowledge in politically and ideologically palatable forms.

Narratives of the evolution of smoking and HIV/AIDS policies in the two European countries make clear the importance of the status of knowledge brokers as recognized experts on health and disease (physicians, medical scientists) and of their position in local medical and scientific hierarchies, either as barriers to or facilitators of the acceptability of public health knowledge. Not only do lay knowledge brokers have little status—and therefore little ability to have their message heard—but also the medical knowledge brokers themselves must be of the right sort.

Among the most consistent themes in accounts of the forces driving tobacco-control policy in Britain is that a *sine qua non* for getting this issue on the government's agenda was the "elite" status of the Royal College of Physicians and of the British Medical Association (which entered the fray in the mid-1980s). Critical to the necessary but delicate political-influence games involved were the access to centers of power and the shared knowledge of appropriate *forms* of action guaranteed both by the social standing of the players (in and outside the world of medicine) and by their preexisting social ties. Similarly, the small group of French physicians behind the initiation of tobacco-control policy in that country were careful to obtain the public adherence of Nobel Prize-winners and other members of the French medical elite. And the opposition of prominent French psychoanalysts was long successful in blocking government sponsorship of measures to prevent HIV/AIDS in injection drug users.

Elite—even scientific—status is a less essential qualification to be a knowledge broker in the United States. In a political culture opposed in principle to hierarchically based authority, experts must take their chances along with everyone else. Political connections and experience in gaming the system are of course valuable in the United States as in Europe, but these resources are less likely to be conferred by elite status, nor are they the exclusive property of old-boy networks. As I have pointed out, nongovernmental brokers of scientific and medical knowledge— including the "zealots" abjured by the British and French—are far more likely to get a hearing in the United Status. Zealous knowledge brokers compete with one another, however, and in the absence of consensus on their relative legitimacy, "fairness" requires that they be given equal time. (The tobacco industry's evaluation of the scientific merits of epidemiologic data on smoking or the National Rifle Association's comments concerning research on gun violence have frequently received as much media attention as the original scientific reports.)[70]

Knowledge brokers must not only have sufficient clout to be heard but also, if they are to be persuasive, must be experts in the framing and interpretation of knowledge in politically and ideologically acceptable forms. In earlier articles I have described "constructions of risk" as a prerequisite to the adoption of public health policies.[71] Credible risks are culturally specific, and knowledge brokers must be culturally as well as scientifically adept at the portrayal of dangers in ways that will galvanize their target audiences. Risk scenarios employed in public health are predictable: dangers are portrayed as being incurred deliberately or involuntarily (and the endangered as correspondingly culpable or innocent), as universal (we are all at risk) or particular (only *they* are at risk), as arising from within the individual or from the environment. The most marketable risks are universal, are attributable to the environment, and are incurred involuntarily.

The meaning and relative importance of these elements are, however, variable across political cultures, as the case studies illustrate. Thus, the "discovery" of risk to the innocent victims of environmental tobacco smoke led to early breakthroughs in U.S. tobacco-control policy, and U.S. tobacco-control advocates have demonstrated a consistent preference for frames that portray smoking as involuntary, the product of immaturity or addiction. Correspondingly, among the obstacles confronted by knowledge brokers in the U.S. AIDS/drugs arena is their inability to make a persuasive case for injection drug use as involuntary or for injection drug users as innocent.[72] While innocent-victim rhetoric is in the toolkits of British and French knowledge brokers as well, it has played a less central role in either tobacco control or AIDS/drugs policy, in part because there is less need to counter the ideology of individual responsibility so ingrained in American audiences.[73]

Scientific and medical data on the dangers of cigarette smoking, on the relative risks of injection drug use as compared with HIV, and on the success of harm minimization programs are equally available in all three countries. Policy differences are not due to uneven access to scientific knowledge. They are due to differences in how—and by whom—these issues are initially framed, to the extent of their politicization, and to differences in the cultural authority of "experts" in the resolution of public health policy issues.

Timing and opportunity contingencies. Timing and opportunity play a critical role in what is or is not held to constitute "knowledge." Passive smoking was accepted as a credible risk in the United States well before any "scientific" evidence of danger, in part because advocates were able to draw on powerful civil rights and environmental frames already in place in the early 1970s. By contrast, although nicotine had long been known to be addictive, framing of smoking as an addiction did not emerge until the mid-1980s. "Old" knowledge of the addictive properties of nicotine was rediscovered and reframed in all three countries, but with somewhat different objectives: in the United States, to bolster the position of tobacco-control advocates and (equally important) of litigators that smoking is not a choice and to further the claims-making of the FDA to regulate tobacco as a drug; in Britain and France, to support the contention of officials, drug treatment experts, and pharmaceutical companies that tobacco control should be treated as a medical rather than as a political problem. Knowledge of nicotine's addictive properties was politically relevant at a later time, whereas it was not relevant earlier.

Similarly, evidence of methadone's value in the treatment of injection drug users did not enter the realm of credible knowledge in France until the AIDS/blood scandal forced the French government to recognize the equally explosive potential of AIDS in injection drug users. Indeed, among the more interesting consequences of the AIDS epidemic is the window of opportunity it created for the emergence of public health as opposed to criminal and/or moral constructions of injection drug use. Experts seized the opportunity with more or less alacrity in all three countries with, as I have observed, varying degrees of success.

Conclusion

An upsurge of concern among American experts in medicine and science about the second Bush administration's "politicization of science" was clearly reflected in comments introducing a recent symposium, "Politics & Science," held at the New School in New York City: "The increasing politicization of science can lead to policy decisions that run counter to accepted scientific consensus and risk endangering our health and well-being."[74] My purpose in this article has been to show that the translation of scientific knowledge into public policy is invariably contingent on an array of social and political forces (including, but not limited to, the discursive practices of scientists themselves) that shift over time and between countries and political cultures. Whatever the dangers to health and well-being, "accepted scientific consensus" (even if it exists) has never been the only player in the policy game.

The contingencies I have described create two major hurdles for scientists to cross. First, they condition whether the statements of experts are—or are not—accepted as authoritative knowledge. Second, they condition whether or not that knowledge becomes the basis for public policy. The former hurdle, I have argued, is particularly formidable in the United States: among the principal strategies employed by opponents of a particular policy is to attack not only the authority of the science on which the policy is based but also the credentials of the experts themselves. The second hurdle is, I suspect, universal. "Policymakers," as Howard Silver points out, "will continue to sort out competing claims and political needs in addition to the scientific evidence to make and implement public policy."[75] And experts will continue to play the political game as well, searching out critical allies, looking for windows of opportunity, framing issues to attract public notice and concern. They have no alternatives if they want their voices heard—and their influence felt—in the cacophonic marketplace of knowledge.

Mailman School of Public Health
Columbia University

Notes

1. In my approach to this analysis I draw on three theoretical traditions, that of the symbolic interactionists, Herbert Blumer, Joseph Gusfield, and others who have written about the construction of public problems: Herbert Blumer, "Social Problems as Collective Behavior," *Social Problems* 18 (1971): 298-307; Joseph R. Gusfield, *The Culture of Public Problems: Drinking-Driving and the Symbolic Order* (Chicago, 1981); Peter Conrad and Joseph W. Schneider, eds., *Deviance and Medicalization: From Badness to Sickness* (St. Louis, 1980); social movement scholars' elaboration of framing processes: David A. Snow, E. Burke Rochford Jr., Steven K. Worden, and Robert D. Benford, "Frame Alignment Process, Micromobilization, and Movement Participation," *American Sociological Review* 51 (1986): 464-81; Doug McAdam, "Culture and Social Movements," in E. Larana, H. Johnston, and J. R. Gusfield, eds., *New Social Movements* (Philadelphia, 1994), 36-57; Sidney Tarrow, *Power in Movement: Social Movements and Contentious Politics*, 2d ed. (Cambridge, 1998); and the work of Mary Douglas and her colleagues and students, who have studied the impact of political cultures on constructions of risks to the environment: Mary Douglas and Aaron Wildavsky, *Risk and Culture: An Essay on the Selection of Technological and Environmental Dangers* (Berkeley and Los Angeles, 1982); Mary Douglas, *Risk and Blame: Essays in Cultural Theory* (London, 1992); Michael Thompson, "Postscript: A Cultural Basis for Comparison," in *Risk Analysis and Decision Processes: The Siting of Liquified Energy Gas Facilities in Four Countries*, ed. Howard C. Kunreuther and Joanne Linerooth, 232-62 (Berlin, 1983); Brian Wynne, *Risk Management and Hazardous Waste: Implementation and the Dialectics of Credibility* (Berlin, 1987). The recent work of Karen Litfin on the science and politics of global environmental risks has been particularly valuable: Karen T. Litfin, *Ozone Discourses: Science and Politics in Global Environmental Cooperation* (New York, 1994).

2. Francois Haas and Sheila Sperber Haas, "The Origins of *Mycobacterium Tuberculosis* and the Notion of Its Contagiousness," in William N. Garay and Stuart M. Rom, eds., *Tuberculosis* (Boston, 1996), 3-19.

3. Pierre Guillaume, *Du Désespoir Au Salut: Les Tuberculeux Aux 19e et 20e Siécles* (Paris, 1986). Villemin's conclusion that tuberculosis was contagious was rejected first in 1865, as I have stated, and again in 1889 (post Koch). Mandatory notification of tuberculosis cases to public health authorities was rejected by the Academy in 1902 and again in 1913. In 1919 mandatory notification was proposed by Premier Georges Clemenceau and was rejected by the National Assembly.

4. Hermann Pidoux (1867), cited in David S. Barnes, *The Making of a Social Disease: Tuberculosis in Nineteenth-Century France* (Berkeley and Los Angeles, 1995), 46.

5. Nowhere (among the four countries I have studied) was mandatory notification uncontested. Nevertheless, New York City implemented notification in 1897 and within ten years eighty-four U.S. cities had followed suit. Notification became law in Britain in 1913.

6. Litfin, *Ozone Discourses*.

7. Intergovernmental Panel on Climate Change (1990), cited in ibid., 193 and 191.

8. The Constance A. Nathanson, *Disease Prevention as Social Change: The State, Society, and Public Health in the U.S., France, Great Britain, and Canada* (New York, 2007).

9. Senator James Inhofe of Oklahoma has gone so far as to claim that "there is scientific evidence that global warming is a 'hoax.'" Cited in Howard J. Silver, "Science and Politics: The Uneasy Relationship," *Open Spaces Quarterly* 8, no. 1 (2005).

10. I have borrowed the useful concept of "knowledge brokers" from Karen Litfin. Knowledge brokers are "intermediaries between the original researchers, or the producers of knowledge, and the policymakers who consume that knowledge but lack the time and training necessary to absorb the original research"(*Ozone Discourses*, 4). Knowledge brokers usually represent state or nonstate agencies or organizations with interests at stake in the matter at hand: civil servants, lobbyists, and activists of various stripes.

11. These case studies are based on detailed interviews with participants in the policy process in each country, on extensive archival research in primary sources, and on the large volume of secondary literature on smoking and HIV/AIDS policies.

12. Royal College of Physicians of London, "Smoking and Health" (London, 1962); U.S. Department of Health, Education, and Welfare, "Smoking and Health: Report of the Advisory Committee to the Surgeon General of the Public Health Service," Public Health Service publication no. 1103 (Washington, D.C., 1964).

13. Brandt comments on the social and cultural meanings attached to the different labels for other people's smoking: "'passive smoking' contrasted with active smoking; 'secondhand smoke' contained the ominous implication that someone else had used it first; involuntary smoking indicated that the practice of smoking was indeed a voluntary act." "Environmental tobacco smoke," or ETS, identifies tobacco smoke as an environmental hazard and, I would add, lends to it the aura of medicine and science attached to other acronyms like STD or DNA. Allan M. Brandt, "Blow Some My Way: Passive Smoking, Risk, and American Culture," in S. Lock, L. A. Reynolds, and E. M. Tansy, eds., *Ashes to Ashes: the History of Smoking and Health* (Amsterdam, 1998), 164–80.

14. Royal College of Physicians of London, "Smoking and Health," S6–7.

15. National Research Council, *Environmental Tobacco Smoke: Measuring Exposures and Assessing Health Effects* (Washington, D.C., 1986); U.S. Department of Health and Human Services, "The Health Consequences of Involuntary Smoking: A Report of the Surgeon General," DHHS publication no. (CDC) 87-8398. U.S. Department of Health and Human Services, Public Health Service, Centers for Disease Control, Center for Health Promotion and Education, Office on Smoking and Health (Rockville, Md., 1986).

16. Virginia Berridge, "Passive Smoking and Its Pre-History in Britain: Policy Speaks to Science?" *Social Science and Medicine* 49 (1999): 1183–95. The "Frogatt report" was the fourth report of the Independent Committee on Smoking and Health, a committee of "scientists and public health interests" appointed in 1973 by then Secretary of State for Health and Social Services, Sir Keith Joseph (ibid., 1187).

17. Maurice Tubiana, "Tabagisme Passif: Rapport et Voeu de L'Académie Nationale de Médicine," *Bulletin de L'Académie Nationale de Médicine* 181, no. 4 (1997): 3–43.

18. See, for example, Richard Kluger, *Ashes to Ashes: America's Hundred-Year Cigarette War, the Public Health, and the Unabashed Triumph of Philip Morris* (New York, 1996). Scientific controversy over the health effects of passive smoking continues to this day. In what was clearly intended as a definitive blow to the credibility of skeptics, Barnes and Bero stated that "the only factor associated with concluding that passive smoking is not harmful was whether an author was affiliated with the tobacco industry." D. E. Barnes and L. Bero, "Why Review Articles on the Health Effects of Passive Smoking Reach Different Conclusions," *Journal of the American Medical Association* 279, no. 19 (1998): 1566–70; 1566. An updated Surgeon General's report on The Health Consequences of Involuntary Exposure to Tobacco Smoke reviews evidence published since 1986 (when the first such report came out) and concludes that "secondhand smoke is a major cause of disease, including lung cancer and coronary heart disease, in healthy nonsmokers" (U.S. Department of Health and Human Services. The Health Consequences of Involuntary Exposure to Tobacco Smoke: A Report to the Surgeon General. Atlanta: U.S. Department of Health and Human Service, Centers for Disease Control and Prevention, Coordinating

Center for Health Promotion, National Center for Chronic Disease Prevention and Health Promotion, Office on Smoking and Health, 2006, i).

19. U.S. Department of Health and Human Services, "Reducing the Health Consequences of Smoking: Twenty-Five Years of Progress. A Report of the Surgeon General," U.S. Department of Health and Human Services publication no. (CDC) 89-8411 (Rockville, Md., 1989), 189.

20. Jesse L. Steinfeld, "Women and Children Last? Attitudes Toward Cigarette Smoking and Nonsmokers' Rights, 1971," *New York State Journal of Medicine* 83, no. 13 (1983): 1257-58; 1258.

21. Unless otherwise noted, all the narrative accounts that follow are drawn from my own research. See, for example, "Social Movements as Catalysts for Policy Change: The Case of Smoking and Guns," *Journal of Health Politics, Policy and Law* 24, no. 3 (1999).

22. *The Ventilator* (1971), 1.

23. The concept of "organizational field," meaning "those organizations that, in the aggregate, constitute a recognized area of institutional life," was introduced by DiMaggio and Powell in 1983: Paul J. DiMaggio and Walter W. Powell, "The Iron Cage Revisited: Institutional Isomorphism and Collective Rationality in Organizational Fields," *American Sociological Review* 48 (April 1983): 148.

24. Clara Gouin, "Nonsmokers and Social Action," Proceedings of the ACS/NCI Conference (DHEW publication no.[NIH] 77-1413), 353-56 (Washington, D.C., 1977), 355.

25. P. Hanauer, G. Barr, and S. Glantz, *Legislative Approaches to a Smoke-Free Society* (Berkeley and Los Angeles, 1986).

26. Kenneth E. Warner, "Cigarette Smoking in the 1970s: The Impact of the Antismoking Campaign," *Science* 211, no. 4483 (1981): 729-31.

27. Ibid., 730.

28. J. Slade, S. A. Glantz, D. E. Barnes, L. Bero, and P. Hanauer, "Nicotine and Addiction: The Brown and Williamson Documents," *Journal of the American Medical Association* 274, no. 3 (1995): 225-33.

29. It is unclear to what extent the smoker-drug addict linkage is accepted by the general public. It is pervasive in public health circles, however, as evidenced by a marked increase over the past decade in the number of articles in the *American Journal of Public Health* associating tobacco with alcohol and drugs, by the naming of an APHA section "Alcohol, tobacco, and other drugs," and by foundation requests for funding applications that link tobacco with narcotic drugs. It is equally popular in legal arguments against the tobacco industry (e.g., Brief for the State of Maryland at 52, *State of Maryland v. Philip Morris et al.*) and in antismoking messages focused on the industry's alleged targeting of children.

30. C. Everett Koop, Preface to "Reducing the Health Consequences of Smoking: Twenty-Five Years of Progress. A Report of the Surgeon General," U.S. Department of Health and Human Services. U.S. Department of Health and Human Services publication no. (CDC) 89-8411 (Rockville, Md., 1989), v.

31. British official publications refer to "passive smoking," the French to "*tabagisme passif.*" Neither countries' publications use a label comparable to the scientific and somewhat more fearsome-sounding "ETS."

32. Roy Porter, "Concluding Remarks," in *Ashes to Ashes*, ed. S. Lock, L. A. Reynolds, and E. M. Tansey, 221-28; David Simpson, "ASH: Witness on Smoking," in *Ashes to Ashes*, ed. S. Lock, L. A. Reynolds, and E. M. Tansey, 208-12.

33. The British aversion to the issue of passive smoking is well illustrated by the fact that in 1985 at the annual meeting of the British Medical Association a motion calling for a Tobacco Act to ban all advertising and sponsorship passed by "a massive majority," while a motion to ban smoking on National Health Service property failed by 20 votes out of 194 on the grounds that such a ban would be cruel to smokers in mental hospitals. British Medical Association, *Smoking Out the Barons: The Campaign Against the Tobacco Industry* (Chichester, 1986), 69.

34. Berridge, "Passive Smoking and Its Pre-History in Britain,"1190. On Valentine's Day 2006, Parliament voted 453 to 125 in favor of a total ban on smoking inside "virtually every enclosed public place and workplace" throughout England. Michael White, "MPs Vote to Stub Out Smoking in Public," *The Guardian*, 24 February 2006, 13. Despite similarities in the discourse around passive smoking, there were striking differences in British as compared to U.S. policy approaches. For example, consistent with the British aversion to legislative regulation, until the newly instituted ban (which will not come into force until the summer of 2007), nonsmoking policies tended to be issued in the form of suggested "guidelines." Furthermore, there was relatively greater emphasis on smoking in the workplace than in spaces open to the public, on the ground that presence in public venues was a matter of choice, whereas presence in the workplace was not. "Indoor Pollution; Restricting Smoking," *British Medical Journal* 303 (1991): 669–70.

35. Note that the "liberty" issue here is not that of nonsmokers to breathe clean air but of smokers to smoke. Nonsmokers are not a significant force in their own right in France. The conflict is not defined as smokers vs. nonsmokers (indeed this is an antagonism that the government and most antitobacco advocates are very concerned to avoid), but the government's responsibility to protect potential victims of involuntary smoking vs. the liberty of smokers.

36. The first paper on the harmful effects of passive smoking generally recognized as being scientifically "authoritative" appeared in the *British Medical Journal* in 1981. T. Hirayama, "Non-Smoking Wives of Heavy Smokers Have a Higher Risk of Lung Cancer: A Study From Japan," *British Medical Journal* 282 (1981): 183–85.

37. Virginia Berridge, "Science and Policy: The Case of Postwar British Smoking Policy," in S. Lock, L. A. Reynolds, and E. M. Tansey, eds., *Ashes to Ashes*, 157.

38. In principle, the incidence of HIV infection would better measure the progress of the epidemic. However, HIV reporting has been highly controversial and has only recently begun to be implemented on any scale. In none of these three countries are reports of HIV infection sufficiently complete or reliable over time to make them useful measures for comparative purposes.

39. Jacques Normand, David Vlahov, and Lincoln E. Moses, *Preventing HIV Transmission: The Role of Sterile Needles and Bleach* (Washington, D.C., 1995).

40. As early as 1986 an elite committee of the National Academy of Sciences, in its first report on the AIDS epidemic, urged the expansion of drug treatment and "experimenting with removing legal barriers to the sale and possession of sterile, disposable needles and syringes." Institute of Medicine/National Academy of Sciences, *Confronting AIDS: Directions for Public Health, Health Care, and Research* (Washington, D.C., 1986).

41. Among the consequences of this construction are, first, to assign primary responsibility for HIV/AIDS in injection drug users to large and bureaucratically powerful drug enforcement and drug treatment bureaucracies. The latter are unsympathetic to any program that assigns priority to disease prevention over the treatment of drug dependence. Second, and not unrelated, designation of HIV/AIDS in injection drug users as a moral issue renders expert "knowledge" irrelevant. Morality policies, as Meier points out, "permit little role for expertise; information that challenges the position of one party or another is often ignored." Kenneth J. Meier, *The Politics of Sin: Drugs, Alcohol, and Public Policy* (Armonk, N.Y., 1994), 4. Federal discountenancing of needle exchange and methadone maintenance has not prevented a range of local initiatives, particularly in the large urban areas most affected by HIV/AIDS.

42. Scottish Home and Health Department, "HIV Infection in Scotland: Report of the Scottish Committee on HIV Infection and Intravenous Drug Misuse," Scottish Home and Health Department (Edinburgh, 1986).

43. Ibid., 4.

44. U.K. Department of Health and Social Security, "AIDS and Drug Misuse: Report by the Advisory Council on the Misuse of Drugs" (London, 1988), 1.

45. Ibid., 2. "Prescribing" in this context refers to the medical prescription of narcotic drugs, primarily-although not limited to-oral methadone.

46. Gerry V. Stimson, "AIDS and Injecting Drug Use in the United Kingdom, 1987–1993: The Policy Response and the Prevention of the Epidemic," *Social Science and Medicine* 41, no. 5 (1995): 699–716; 704. "Pilot" is in quotes because this designation was intended to take the heat off arguments against syringe exchange. "We knew they really weren't," commented a civil servant intimately involved with this activity at the time. Exchange of sterile for used needles and syringes is labeled "syringe-exchange" in Britain. In the United States, "needle" and "syringe" exchange are used interchangeably.

47. J. Parsons, M. Hickman, P. Turnball, T. McSweeney, G. V. Stimson, A. Judd, and K. Roberts, "Over a Decade of Syringe Exchange: Results from 1997 UK Survey," *Addiction* 97, no. 7 (2002): 845–50; 845. Syringe-exchange programs were a major policy innovation. To complete the picture of HIV-prevention facilities available to injection-drug users in Britain, it is important to point out that there are no legal barriers either to over-the-counter sales of syringes or to the prescription of oral or injectable methadone.

48. Susanne MacGregor, "The Public Debate in the 1980s," in Susanne MacGregor, ed., *Drugs and British Society* (London, 1989).

49. John Street and Albert Weale, "Britain: Policy-Making in a Hermetically Sealed System," in David L. Kirp and Ronald Bayer, eds., *AIDS in the Industrialized Democracies: Passions, Politics, and Policies* (New Brunswick, N.J., 1992), 185–220.

50. Gerry V. Stimson and Rachel Lart, "The Relationship Between the State and Local Practice in the Development of National Policy on Drugs Between 1920 and 1990," in J. Strang, and M. Gossop, eds., *Heroin Addiction and Drug Policy: The British System* (Oxford, 1994), 331–41.

51. "Ultimately," Berridge observes, "both the tabloid press and public opinion had no effect on policy." Virginia Berridge, "AIDS, the Media and Health Policy," *Health Education Journal* 50, no. 4 (1991): 184.

52. My account of French drug treatment professionals' ideology and its implications for their confrontation with AIDS is based on published sources and on my interviews with several of the actors involved. Published sources include: Anne Coppel, "Les Intervenants en Toxicomanie, le Sida et la Réduction des Risques en France," in *Vivre avec les Drogues* (Paris, 1996), 75–108; Alain Ehrenberg, *L'Individu Incertain* (Paris, 1995); Roger Henrion, *Rapport de la Comission de Réflexion sur la Drogue et la Toxicomanie* (Paris, 1995); Emile Malet, ed., *Santé Publique et Libertés Individuelles* (Paris, 1993).

53. It may be worth noting that the job of public health authorities is made easier when disease prevention and drug-use prevention are synonymous, as in the case of tobacco smoking. "Safe" drug use is a harder sell.

54. French drug treatment specialists had a particular horror of what they saw as "American-style" methadone maintenance programs, requiring daily visits for medication and monitoring of patients' urine to ensure compliance. It is striking that these specialists found it far easier to accept syringe exchange-which they saw as an autonomous act by the drug user-than methadone maintenance, which (in their eyes) implicated the physician in the user's actions. At least one prominent drug-treatment specialist suggested that it might be preferable to sell methadone like cigarettes than for it to be prescribed.

55. The quote is from my interview with a longtime civil servant in the drug policy arena.

56. The point was frequently called to my attention that two figures who played a major role in shifting France's drugs policies in response to HIV/AIDS, Michelle Barzach and Simone Veil, were both on the Right.

57. Among many examples of and reflections on this ideological perspective, see the compilation of articles and brief statements from a symposium titled *Santé publique et libertés individuelles* and a lengthy interview with Claude Got that appeared in *Le Monde* on 17 June 1992.

58. Monika Steffen, "France: Social Solidarity and Scientific Expertise," in David L. Kirp and Ronald Bayer, eds., *AIDS in the Industrialized Democracies: Passions, Politics, and Policies* (New Brunswick, N.J., 1992), 221–51; Aquilino Morelle, *La Défaite de la Santé Publique* (Paris, 1996).

59. Mary Douglas, *Risk and Blame*, 32.

60. Sheila Jasanoff, "American Exceptionalism and the Political Acknowledgment of Risk," *Daedalus* (Fall 1990): 61-81; 76.

61. Stephen G. Brint, *In an Age of Experts: The Changing Role of Professionals in Politics and Public Life* (Princeton, 1994), 200.

62. Brian Wynne, *Risk Management and Hazardous Waste*, 421.

63. Decisions to appoint a committee of the "great and the good" and the choice of committee members are not, of course, made in a political vacuum, nor are the deliberations and decisions of these committees apolitical. For an excellent account of their use to suppress and distort "knowledge" in the case of mad cow disease, see: David. Miller, "Risk, Science and Policy: Definitional Struggles, Information Management, the Media and BSE," *Social Science and Medicine* 49 (1999): 1239-55.

64. Brint, *In an Age of Experts*, 195.

65. Ezra N. Suleiman, *Elites in French Society: The Politics of Survival* (Princeton, 1978), 4.

66. Michèle Lamont, *Money, Morals, and Manners: The Culture of the French and American Upper-Middle Class* (Chicago, 1992).

67. Bruno Jobert, "Mobilisation Politique et Système de Santé en France," in *Les Politiques de Santé en France et en Allemagne*, ed. Bruno Jobert and Monika Steffen, 73-81 (Paris, 1994).

68. See, for example, Eric A. Feldman and Ronald Bayer, eds., *Blood Feuds: AIDS, Blood, and the Politics of Medical Disaster* (New York, 1999).

69. Litfin, *Ozone Discourses*, 37.

70. It is a measure of the tobacco-control movement's success in the United States that, at least in recent years, the tobacco industry has largely disappeared from the media as a credible source on questions of smoking and health.

71. Constance A. Nathanson, "Disease Prevention as Social Change: Toward a Theory of Public Health," *Population and Development Review* 22, no. 4 (1996): 609-37; "Social Movements as Catalysts for Policy Change: The Case of Smoking and Guns," *Journal of Health Politics, Policy and Law* 24, no. 3 (1999).

72. One of many paradoxes in a comparison between American society's current constructions of nicotine and heroin as addictive drugs is the relatively benign connotation of "addiction" in the former as compared to the latter case.

73. This difference in the importance of "innocent victim" rhetoric is strikingly reflected in American and French legal briefs against the tobacco industry. A major reason for plaintiffs' failure to recover in U.S. tobacco litigation until very recently was that individuals who became sick from smoking were regarded as responsible for their own fate. Claimants simply did "not qualify as 'deserving' victims." Robert A. Kagan and David Vogel, "The Politics of Smoking Regulation: Canada, France, the United States," *Smoking Policy: Law, Politics, and Culture*, ed. Robert L. Rabin and Stephen D. Sugarman, 22-48 (New York, 1994), 126. Given this history, plaintiffs' tobacco litigation experts were understandably concerned that individuals bringing suit be portrayable, and be portrayed, as "innocent" of responsibility for their claimed injuries. Richard A. Daynard, "Catastrophe Theory and Tobacco Litigation," *Tobacco Control* 3 (1994): 62. In France, the state, through its official organs, determined that smoking was a danger to the public's health. The guilt or innocence of smoking victims was simply not a legally cognizable issue. More generally, "fault" has a relatively attenuated role in the French equivalent of tort law but is central to legal determinations of guilt or innocence in the United States.

74. The New School, "Science & Politics." Web page, February 2006 [accessed 10 March 2006]. Available at http://www.socres.org/polsci; see also Howard J. Silver, "Science and Politics: The Uneasy Relationship," *Open Spaces Quarterly* 8, no. 1 (2005).

75. Silver, "Science and Politics" (n.p.). Silver has been the executive director of COSSA (Consortium of Social Science Associations), the principal lobbying group for social science, since 1988.

HAROLD POLLACK

Learning to Walk Slow: America's Partial Policy Success in the Arena of Intellectual Disability

The history of policies affecting individuals with intellectual disabilities has received attention from social historians interested in gender and family, from the emerging discipline of disability studies, and from scholars interested in the evolving role of eugenic arguments and medical genetics in American life. That history has received less systematic study from the community of policy analysts and scholars traditionally concerned with welfare, poverty, and public health. This is unfortunate because the history of policies affecting intellectual disability offers at least three significant lessons.

First, this history underscores the role of compassion as a valuable but ambiguous political asset for mobilizing resources. Most existing accounts, including James Trent's essential *Inventing the Feeble Mind*, emphasize the influence of class ideologies, racial antagonism, eugenics, family, and gender roles in shaping public policies, clinical interventions, and social norms regarding persons living with cognitive disabilities.[1] In a more specialized study, Paul Castellani emphasizes the importance of political economy, tracing out the intricacies of institutional closure and Medicaid policy that affected immediate stakeholders.[2] Neither of these studies captures the distinctive role played by persons with intellectual disability and their caregivers, or the interplay between the social politics of intellectual disability and the intricate web of institutions and interventions that serve these citizens and their families. While interest-group politics, narrowly construed, can help analysts understand why

This article is the beginning of a broader project. The editor and Eileen Boris provided valuable comments.

public sector unions might try to protect jobs in institutional care, it cannot explain the dramatic shift from institutional to community-based care. Nor can it explain why federal, state, and local expenditures on services for intellectual disability have strongly increased over decades. Traditional interest-group politics cannot explain successful litigation that changed the face of American education, health care, and workplace to embrace disabled persons or the remarkably broad acceptance of the Americans with Disabilities Act (ADA), a complex, costly, and often burdensome federal law enacted under a Republican administration.

The intellectually disabled are often depicted in a disparaging light, most recently and frankly in *The Bell Curve*. Yet from *Pilgrim's Progress* to *Forest Gump* and *Life Goes On*,[3] disparaging images have coexisted with sympathetic portrayals that bring different resonances for public policy.[4] Aside from dramatic imagery, fiscal accounting reveals the latent generosity of an American welfare state that draws stark distinctions among recipients of public help. The same society that stigmatizes millions of people deemed unworthy of help proves surprisingly generous toward those, such as intellectually disabled persons, it deems in genuine need of help. The same history suggests that compassion can bring its own ambiguous implications in framing policy debate. Appeals to compassion help to elicit public resources for custodial care and treatment to keep persons with intellectual disabilities clean, safe, and healthy. Such appeals do not elicit sustained efforts to address more complex, multi-faceted challenges faced by disabled persons.

Second, this history underscores the role of family caregivers as political actors and as specific objects of public concern. A key political dilemma of traditional AFDC was that voters and policymakers wished to help low-income children but seemed unhappy about the prospect of subsidizing the unmarried mothers with whom most such children lived.[5] No such dilemmas arose in intellectual disability. Drawn from a broad cross section of society, family caregivers have been performing an honored, increasingly public role. Drawn together by exigencies of educational, health, and social services, mobilized by organizations such as ARC, caregivers marshaled impressive political resources to advance their interests at every level of government.

Third, the policy history of intellectual disability underscores inherent limitations of the American welfare state in serving even those distinctive groups it wishes to treat well. Persons living with intellectual disabilities and their families receive more generous funding and services than do other groups. Yet they encounter obstacles imposed by means-tested programs, decentralized interventions that receive limited bureaucratic direction or oversight, and age-based interventions that are often ill-suited to the needs of intellectually disabled adults.

For persons with intellectual disability and their caregivers, policy history provides reason for optimism because it reveals how far the United States has come. As recently as 1900, emerging genetic science supported strategies to minimize perceived social burdens imposed by disabled persons and to manage the human gene pool. Eugenic interest spanned the political spectrum. Charles Eliot Norton, among others, proposed "painless destruction" of those with mental disabilities.[6] When the *Journal of the American Medical Association* published the nation's first report of vasectomy, the author noted the procedure's utility for "chronic inebriates, imbeciles, perverts and paupers," along with "racial degeneracy."[7]

Attitudes shifted during the 1940s, a decade that marked the emergence of both family and institutional caregiving as topics for discussion in popular culture. Before then, shame and stigma generally precluded open discussion of such intimate concerns. Indeed, the intensity of social pressure—combined with a fear that the burdens of caregiving would unduly harm other family members—had pushed many parents to covertly institutionalize a child, sometimes without even revealing that the child was born. Such decisions crossed economic and educational lines. In 1944, Eric and Joan Erickson had a child diagnosed with Down's syndrome. The Ericksons concealed the child from their other children, saying that he had died at birth.[8]

Not surprisingly, everyday realities of institutional care were also kept far from public view.[9] World War II helped change that, partly in response to Nazi policies, partly because of wartime exigencies that led conscientious objectors to be detailed to state institutions for the retarded. Idealistic and often highly educated, many of those conscripts were horrified by what they saw. Some wrote about their experiences, sparking a postwar wave of public exposés of institutional care. A 1946 article in *Christian Century* received national attention for its frank portrayal of the brutal and unsanitary conditions at one large underfunded state facility.[10]

The 1940s also marked passage of the National Mental Health Act and the founding of the National Institute of Mental Health. The NIMH budget was initially modest, with only a small portion devoted to intellectual disability.[11] Yet spending increased rapidly. New legislation solidified a federal role in research and funding for services to persons with intellectual disability. In 1954, President Eisenhower declared the first National Retarded Children's Week. Between 1956 and 1961, pertinent federal funding increased from $14 million to $94 million.[12]

The supposedly conservative 1950s also marked structural expansions in federal income support to disabled persons. In 1950, federal policymakers amended the Social Security Act to authorize payments to "Permanently and Totally Disabled" persons. Legislation in 1956 guaranteed Social Security aid to the "Disabled Adult Children" (DAC) of deceased, retired, or disabled Social Security recipients.[13] DAC provided one key pillar of entitlement security for persons living with disability. It would take another Republican administration, in 1972, to create the other pillar, Supplemental Security Income (SSI).[14] The divide between policy scholarship and disability studies is reflected in the fact that few historical studies of intellectual disability include specific discussion of these key income-support programs.[15]

In 1950 Pearl Buck published *The Child Who Never Grew*, becoming the first celebrity to openly relate her experience as the mother of a retarded daughter.[16] The only American woman to win both Nobel and Pulitzer prizes, Buck had a huge readership. First in the pages of *Ladies' Home Journal*, later as a short best-selling book, *The Child Who Never Grew* broke taboos by recounting Buck's gradual discovery of her daughter Carolyn's disability, Buck's struggle to accept the severity and permanence of Carolyn's cognitive limitations and finally the difficult decision to institutionalize Carolyn at the noted Training School in Vineland, New Jersey.

The Child Who Never Grew sparked interest and sympathy among millions of readers. It spawned a noteworthy affirmational literature by parents in similar straits, most notably Dale Evans's 1953 best-selling account, *Angel Unaware*.[17] These works helped temper fear and stigma directed at persons, particularly children, living with intellectual disabilities. In doing so, these books engaged and reinforced cultural narratives that remain central to disability policy debate. They frankly chronicled the struggle facing even privileged parents who sought to accept and understand the reality of their child's condition, obtain basic services, and create long-term arrangements that would ensure reliable and attentive care after they themselves were gone.

By emphasizing the helpless innocence of cognitively disabled persons, such books grounded caregiving discourse in redemptive Christian charity. In these narratives, persons with intellectual disabilities required simple vocational training, combined with safe and loving custodial care. The authors stressed the importance of prevention science—an effort that would bear fruit with the discovery of treatments for PKU. They paid scant attention to what would now be called services research, and generally downplayed the individuality and varied circumstances over the life course of actual persons with disability. While noting the many challenges families encountered, and sometimes offering advice about medical and educational concerns, these memoirists presented caregiving as a private tragedy and burden to be managed rather than as an explicit domain for public policy intervention.

As Janice Brockey notes, an undertone of guilt and unease is readily apparent in these accounts.[18] Like other memoirists of the time, Pearl Buck sought to explain and justify her decision to institutionalize Carolyn at nine years of age. "I realized then that I must find another world for my child, one where she would not be despised and rejected, one where she could find her own level and have friends and affection."

Buck recounted a visit to the Mayo Clinic, which she visited during her early search for explanations regarding Carolyn's cognitive problems. After Carolyn's pediatric examination was over, an unfamiliar doctor beckoned her to an adjoining room:

> "Did he tell you the child might be cured?" He demanded.
> "He—he didn't say she could not," I stammered.
> "Listen to what I tell you," he commanded. "I tell you, madame. The child will never be normal. Do not deceive yourself. You will wear out your life and beggar your family unless you give up hope and face the truth. . . . Above all, do not let her absorb you. Find a place where she can be happy and live your own life." (43)

Buck responded surprisingly to this unsolicited and ferocious assessment: "I shall always be grateful to him, whose name I do not even know. He cut the wound deep, but it was clean and quick. I was brought at once face to face with the inevitable."

Perhaps Buck embellished this odd encounter, but as James Trent first observed, other memoirs of the period recount similar incidents, in which professionals bluntly recommended institutionalization as the only possible course.[19] A 1955 story, "Unfit Mother," goes so far as to rebuke a mother who refuses to institutionalize her disabled son, thereby neglecting her husband and other children.[20] Parents were expected to defer to professional care. Professionals, in turn, were expected to ease parents' guilt and pain by emphasizing the necessity of institutional care.

The Child Who Never Grew can be jarring when judged by today's norms. Like other parents in the same situation, Buck noted her strong family stock. She pointedly denied that Carolyn suffered from genetic disability, saying, "The old stigma of 'something in the family' is all too often unjust." Such denials issued at the dawn of the genetic era were often misplaced. Carolyn actually suffered from PKU, now a readily treated genetic disorder.

The book's title bespeaks a focus on her daughter. Yet the dominant story concerned Pearl Buck herself—her insights and accomplishments, grief, and struggles as she cared for her daughter. Her estranged husband and her other (adopted) children are not mentioned. Carolyn herself, especially in her teen and later years, is often invisible or described in generic terms. Buck never mentions Carolyn's name.

The 1992 re-release of *The Child Who Never Grew* included an afterword by Buck's daughter Janice Walsh. One must consult this affecting essay to glean basic family details. Walsh makes plain that Pearl Buck's driving ambition cast some dark shadows over family life. Buck wrote more than one hundred books. She accomplished much in her charity work. She loved her children. Yet her rich intellectual and political life made her a distant presence. Walsh writes that Pearl dreamed of "making amends to her children." She adds, "This magnificent woman—my mother—left a legacy that could not be duplicated, but she also left lives that would need healing."

Love and worry for Carolyn spurred Buck's frenetic productivity, but Buck was not prepared to provide the relentless care Carolyn required. Caring for someone with cognitive disability is hard under the best of circumstances. Not every parent can or should assume this task. Perhaps fearing that her audience would judge her harshly, Buck did not acknowledge this painful reality. She had much at stake in convincing the reader that the only alternative to institutionalizing her daughter was for she herself to assume superhuman burdens. A later, more intimate genre of caregiving accounts would more frankly discuss the intimate trade-offs caregivers confront, as we balance our efforts to help a disabled loved one with our desire to help others we love and to pursue our own lives.[21]

Buck also echoed a long-standing notion articulated by the governor of Massachusetts as early as 1884: "A well-fed idiot, well-cared-for idiot is a happy creature. An idiot awakened to his condition is a miserable one."[22] For this reason and others, Buck asserted that people with intellectual disability are happiest among people "like themselves." Charlotte Tucker, in *Betty Lee*, expressed similar views. Noting that children with disabilities "cannot compete with the normal group," she forthrightly argued that they be protected from resulting hurtful experiences. The perceived fear that persons with intellectual disabilities will discover and be crushed by their predicament, and the related belief that it is possible to protect them from the central reality of their lives, provided powerful motivation for social isolation and for institutional care.

Titles such as *The Child Who Never Grew* served another key purpose. They framed intellectual disability as a matter of parents caring for their children. Writers like Buck, and their readers, were surely comforted to regard adults with intellectual disabilities as children, angels unaware. Experts and lay people routinely spoke of "mental age" and deployed other language with similar connotations. In some obvious ways, metaphorical links between intellectual disability and childhood matched the perception and the reality of family care. Images of childlike innocence proved a powerful metaphor to elicit public sympathy and support, and to undercut pervasive public fears. It neatly sidestepped widespread anxieties regarding sexuality and reproduction among men and women with intellectual disabilities.[23]

This vocabulary and rhetoric was suited to the times in which these books were read. Statistical realities provided one reason for treating intellectually disabled persons as a population of children. Through the 1950s, many persons with intellectual disabilities died in childhood or before their early twenties. Improved survival has been most dramatic for Down's syndrome, which is often accompanied by cardiac complications that once routinely caused premature death. In 1929, mean lifespan for an infant born with Down's syndrome was nine years. By the 1990s, life expectancy of a one-year-old child with Down's syndrome and mild/moderate retardation had reached fifty-five years, and is still rising.[24]

Aside from the epidemiology, postwar American culture provided unusual opportunities and requirements for parents, especially mothers, to politically mobilize on behalf of their children with intellectual disabilities. A detailed history of these matters has yet to be written. However, existing research already delineates key features of this history, particularly in two essays by Kathleen W. Jones and Katherine Castles.[25]

Jones and Castles cite postwar middle-class familialism in the development of the National Association of Retarded Children (NARC). Within this cultural frame, mothers enjoyed political space to advocate for educational and social advancement of their disabled children. Parents faced the pressing need for normalizing experiences such as summer camp and beach vacations. Children with intellectual disabilities posed a threat to domesticity. The intense time demands of caregiving could prevent mothers from meeting their other children's (and their husbands') needs. Traditional family values thus ironically encouraged parents to seek institutional care.

Jones profiles the local activism of New Jersey housewife Laura Blossfeld, who helped to found what would become the New Jersey Parents Group for Retarded Children. In 1946, Blossfeld placed an advertisement in a Bergen County newspaper recruiting other parents to join the nascent organization. Her pitch might have been drawn from a political science textbook: "Each parent can ultimately help his own child by doing something to help all children similarly affected. . . . Therefore I suggest an organization for all parents of mentally retarded children, [one that] may well prove to be the first chapter in a nationwide organization." Other activists made similar appeals. In 1949, a New York City housewife placed a similar newspaper advertisement, writing, "Surely there must be other children like [her son], other parents like myself. Where are you? Let's band together and *do something* for our children!"[26]

By 1950, Blossfeld's northern New Jersey group had expanded to seven chapters. In 1952, parent groups in many states mobilized to form the National Association for Retarded Children (NARC). Proceeds from *Angel Unaware* provided NARC's first major donation.[27] An internal history relates NARC's explosive early growth.[28] By 1955, NARC had 412 local affiliates and 29,000 members. Some 296 chapters offered direct services to members, nursery school classes, recreational and social groups, parent counseling, and social welfare referrals. In addition to direct service delivery, NARC chapters established local lobbying groups and provided or subsidized training for service providers. By 1960, NARC had 681 local affiliates and 62,000 members. By 1964, membership topped 100,000. NARC quickly acquired influence, working closely with congressional allies and with several presidential administrations.

Mindful of the stigma associated with intellectual disability, NARC sought to change public perceptions. Its materials emphasized that intellectual disability crosses racial, economic, and class lines. This rhetoric elided some disparities in the actual incidence of intellectual disability. Nor did NARC's inclusive rhetoric reflect its own membership. A 1974 survey indicated that 96 percent of NARC members were white. Most were married, had attended college, and reported middle-class incomes.[29] But NARC's avowedly universal message allowed advocates for intellectually disabled persons to sidestep economic and racial antagonisms that might otherwise stymie efforts to secure public resources.

As both Jones and Castles recount, NARC's agenda, vocabulary, and rhetoric reflected mothers' initial dominance within the organization. NARC was also politically active, promoting what would become special education and supporting state bond issues to expand residential treatment. During the 1960s, NARC became a key member of the "mind lobby," advocating the expansion of community-based mental health and mental retardation services. The "mind lobby" proved remarkably potent. As David Felicetti put it, "The mind lobbies . . . confront[ed] virtually no political enemies in Congress" (124). Edward Berkowitz and others document NARC's (and its successors') continuing influence in Reagan-era disability policy reforms (145–46).[30]

NARC's long-term efforts are reflected in the two most prominent federal laws affecting citizens with intellectual disabilities: the Americans with Disabilities Act (ADA) and Public Law 94–142, the Education for All Handicapped Children Act. Both measures, despite political and legal challenges, remain popular. In a 2003 Harris survey, more than 85 percent of Americans supported laws barring discrimination against the disabled in employment and in public accommodations. More than three-quarters favored laws requiring "reasonable accommodations for employees with disabilities" by large and midsize firms.[31] Ratifying and expressing this consensus, court decisions such as *Olmstead v. L.C.* altered the landscape of community and institutional care, while cases such as *PARC v. Commonwealth of Pennsylvania*,[32] and *Sullivan v. Zebley* redefined the educational and social service entitlements available to intellectually disabled children.[33]

Media images of the intellectually disabled, once dominated by fearful or freakish imagery, increasingly include recognizably sympathetic individuals, many living with mild or moderate cognitive disabilities and who successfully accomplish work, school, and family roles. Major newspapers routinely present stories about the everyday lives of persons with intellectual disabilities: their dating and work lives, their dilemmas in school.[34]

By 2004, 1.2 million Americans from eighteen to sixty-four received Social Security or SSI benefits due to qualifying diagnoses of intellectual disability.[35] Such transfers provided the financial foundation for a real, if incomplete, transition from institutional to community-based care. The quality, intensity, and range of services offered to persons with intellectual disability have sharply increased. Coincident with these trends, average lifespan and health status of persons with intellectual disability have also risen. Inflation-adjusted expenditures for community-based intellectual disability services have increased by 10 percent annually since 1977.[36] By 2004, public spending for community and institution-based care reached $38.5 billion,[37] exceeding the $28.5 billion spent by states and the federal government for Temporary Assistance to Needy Families. This $38.5 billion figure does not include many other sources of aid, including special education, food stamps, and cash assistance, flowing to intellectually disabled persons.

The political position of family caregivers also changed. In 1950, family caregivers were politically disorganized. Over time, however, the evolution of NARC reflected and spurred the rise of family caregivers as a self-conscious constituency. In this manner, NARC differed in several ways from other voluntary associations of the late twentieth century, such as the March of Dimes. Lay NARC leadership resisted domination by physicians, mental health professionals, or representatives from service agencies. NARC parents kept their challenges and frustrations at the forefront of their activities in schools, hospitals, and social service systems. Those priorities were crisply expressed in a 1959 essay by Mrs. Max Murray, chairwoman of the Virginia Association for Retarded Children.[38] In an article, "Needs of Parents of Mentally Retarded Children," published in the flagship *American Journal of Mental Deficiency*, Murray identified six basic problems parents faced:

1. Acceptance of the fact that a child is retarded.
2. Emotional burdens, aggravated by the inability to share these burdens with others.
3. The challenge to religious faith facing families who have often experienced tragedy.
4. Financial burdens imposed by intellectual disability.
5. The need to provide love, guidance, and care beyond the lifetime of the current caregiver.
6. Coping with inept, inaccurate, or ill-timed professional advice.

Murray boldly and presciently emphasized this last point. She noted that medical, educational, and social service professionals sometimes lacked "emotional and spiritual maturity," and thus provided inferior care. She provided specific examples in which teachers, pediatricians, and psychiatrists provided incorrect, poorly communicated, misleading, or wrongly paternalistic advice to parents, with detrimental results. She noted that parents who appeared "defensive" may adopt this stance because of "a former unfortunate contact with an emotionally immature and insecure professional person." Anticipating a later generation of patient advocates, Mrs. Murray commented: "*The greatest single need of parents of mentally retarded children is constructive professional counseling at various stages in the child's life which will enable the parents to find the answers to their own individual problems*" (emphasis in original).

Such accounts marked the beginning of a new assertiveness, a transformation of family care from a private activity performed under professional guidance to an organized, avowedly public role. If professionals require monitoring, if their commitment, maturity, and expertise could not be fully trusted, family caregivers required their own sources of information and expertise. If medical, educational, and social service providers were unwilling to provide needed accommodations, families needed procedures to state their case. They needed the leverage to ensure that their case would be heard. It would take more than a decade for these ideas to be codified in PL 94–142, but the basic sensibility was there.

The scale of social change is ironically revealed by the changing self-presentation of NARC itself. For twenty years, NARC's logo depicted a child and the stark statement: "Retarded children can be helped." Originally founded as the National Association of Parents and Friends of Mentally Retarded Children, it changed its name in 1973 to the National Association of Retarded Citizens. In 1981, it was again renamed to ARC, Association of Retarded Citizens. In 1992, it became simply the Arc, whose name corresponds to no specified initials.[39]

In 1950, as today, mothers provided the dominant share of family support for intellectually disabled persons. Cohort analyses indicate that more than 90 percent of intellectually disabled adults who live with relatives live with their parents; very few transition into permanent arrangements with siblings or other relatives.[40] NARC and related groups were thus dominated by mothers seeking services, economic security, and social acceptance for their children. Mothers' focus on children proved especially important in defining and financing special educational services, which were a central battleground for many parents. Despite mandatory attendance laws, children with intellectual disabilities were often barred from public schools, which lacked the resources or expertise to serve them.[41] Exclusion deprived children of educational resources and deprived parents of support and respite from care.

The focus on children brought less-noticed but problematic implications for policy and for public discourse. NARC's focus on children obscured pressing issues that faced the growing majority of intellectually disabled persons in the United States, who were and remain adults. An approach that centered on mothers and children also tended to frame schools (rather than, say, housing or medical care) as the natural domain of public intervention. But because the state's obligations to provide a free and appropriate education end in the late teens, thousands of men and women confronted the quandary of "aging out" of traditional schooling every year.[42]

A second pressing issue concerned intergenerational transitions in caregiving. By 2004, an estimated 711,000 Americans with intellectual disability lived with caregivers over the age of sixty.[43] Many were able to live with their parents due to federal income support policies that provided a financial foundation for home-based care. They now face a difficult transition into alternative arrangements as their parents retire, become disabled themselves, or die.[44]

This last challenge underscored deeper obstacles that NARC confronted. As advocates for a specific group, NARC used grassroots advocacy to leverage distinctive public concerns for intellectually disabled citizens. It operated, however, within the existing grooves of a fragmented welfare state that is poorly equipped to address chronic disability over the life course. NARC could fight for incremental changes to particular interventions that improved services for specific constituents—as it successfully did for children. But it could do little to improve the nation's patchwork of overlapping programs, operated and funded across different levels of government.

Joseph Soss has found that public assistance has the potential to politically empower or marginalize aid recipients.[45] He found that interactions with Social Security disability programs bolstered clients' sense of equal citizenship, while recipients' interactions with AFDC had quite opposite effects. Citizens with intellectual disabilities and their caregivers have both kinds of experiences. They enjoy secure, well-funded federal entitlements applied across the country. They simultaneously encounter the vagaries of state and local programs that vary in generosity, eligibility requirements, and operational performance. Families encounter waiting lists for sheltered workshops and group homes. Those services, nonentitlements, languish in many communities. By 2003, 51,000 persons with intellectual disabilities were on formal state waiting lists for residential services.[46]

Most Americans living with significant intellectual disabilities receive Medicaid,[47] the dominant and often only payer for key services. Few families, even among the affluent, could provide care without it. So they do what they legally can to maintain eligibility. States recognize these realities by establishing (or tolerating) asset-shielding arrangements. Many families are nonetheless forced to resort to backhanded strategies that create unforeseen complications. Some nominally disinherit a disabled child, leaving funds to an able-bodied sibling who is honor-bound to help. These arrangements have no legal force, and they create new difficulties. Some able-bodied siblings die or divorce. Others borrow funds intended for their sibling.[48]

Caregivers face the challenge of monitoring the quality and performance of decentralized services. Community-based residential care is provided through 140,000 group homes and other settings. Despite efforts at accreditation, there is no systematic way for caregivers to evaluate a specific setting against well-defined standards of care.[49] Adding to caregivers' anxiety, the basic capacity of policymakers to detect and address blatantly substandard care remains unclear.[50]

Families encounter contradictory rules and procedures at different levels of government, which complicate efforts at long-term planning. Thus, an individual with Down's syndrome who lives with his mother effectively enjoys a lifetime entitlement to Social Security and Medicare that is unaffected by his location or financial assets. These payments are generally channeled through a representative payee who is responsible to account for the money but is never queried about much else. When caregivers die, persons with disability face the loss of Medicaid if they inherit assets or if they must cross state lines to establish new living arrangements.

Programmatic discordance arises from the division of labor across levels of government, which affects favored and disfavored groups alike. Courts can sometimes smooth these gaps or enforce welfare rights.[51] They are less effective in creating strong administrative structures or in expanding the pool of available resources for costly interventions.[52]

For people who wish to be recognized for their individual identities as equal citizens, compassion carries an especially high price when it depicts adults as needy children. Although children and parents have distinct interests, traditional American social insurance (although not traditional welfare) helps children by helping their parents. Viewing adults with intellectual disabilities as children draws scant attention to the possibility that they might have different interests and priorities from those expressed by their parents or other caregivers.

Over the past half-century, the United States has done much to embrace citizens with intellectual disabilities. Caregivers and their allies created a political foundation for public action and achieved concrete victories that improved quality of life for intellectually disabled persons and their families. These victories included expanded entitlements to cash aid, vast expansion in public funding for community-based services, and laws and court decisions that recognized the rights of intellectually disabled persons in education, health care, and transportation. These victories also included profound change in social practice outside the domain of explicit public policy. Life goes on very differently from before. Early memoirs of caregiving describe a bygone world.

Memoirists who exposed their intimate and tragic struggles to public view, and the parent-founders of NARC whom they inspired, were not the only important actors in bringing about these profound policy shifts. The Kennedy administration and family, legal advocates, and a later generation of disability activists also played key roles.[53] Yet these early actors remain important. If they sometimes lacked the language or vision to honor their children's predicament, their work spurred policies that moved beyond where they themselves had been.

Theda Skocpol writes in *Protecting Soldiers and Mothers:*

> Institutional arrangements and electoral rules . . . affect which of the society's groups become active in politics, and when. Given that certain groups do become politically active, moreover, some of them achieve more political leverage than others. Much of the reason has to do with the "fit," or lack thereof, between a nation's governing institutions at a given time and the goals and organizational capacities of the various groups and alliances that seek to influence policymaking.[54]

Skocpol laments the declining political potency of maternalist ideals in U.S. social policy. She describes advocates as increasingly privileged and insulated, operating from foundations, universities, or public-interest law firms, speaking in specialized discourse, economically and socially distant from those they seek to help. "These fine people," she writes, "defend and promote anti-poverty programs that no longer arise from an encompassing movement with broad appeal across the population of politically active American women" (537). She writes that "U.S. advocates for mothers and children are *not* supported by federations that regularly reach from the great urban centers down to local communities across the entire nation."

In one way, the history of intellectual disability challenges Skocpol's pessimistic views. Over a period in which mothers and children were specifically deprived of federal cash entitlements, public provision to intellectually disabled persons retained broad political support. Intellectually disabled persons won legal victories that expanded their rights to education, cash aid, and institutional care.[55] As scholars debated why welfare states retrench, America continued to expand large and costly maternalist programs for millions of intellectually disabled persons.

This expansion reflects precisely the political opportunities available to groups in position to follow Skocpol's advice. With surprising speed, NARC's founders created a large national federation of organizations, dominated by women, which would alter the social politics of intellectual disability. NARC members recognized the necessity of government action to meet their needs. They recognized the need for collective action to enact these policies.

For many Americans, the childlike innocence readily identified with cognitive disability exemplified our image of worthy persons who need and deserve help. NARC campaigns featured endorsements by Earl Warren and other prominent Americans. The cause of intellectual disability has continued to attract support from affluent and educated citizens across political lines. When officials in the Reagan administration sought to curtail PL 94–142, they were opposed by Republican Senator Lowell Weicker and conservative columnist George Will, each caring for a son with Down's syndrome.[56] NARC and its successors were spared race and class antagonisms that animate other policy debates.

So persons with intellectual disability and their families have experienced some of the best our welfare state can offer. Yet our genuine efforts to help reveal inherent limitations in what our welfare state actually provides. Persons with intellectual disabilities benefit from their distinctive appeal, from grassroots pressures to specifically respond to their needs. These assets do not protect them against defects in the existing structures through which we provide public aid. Some structures, such as the DAC program, effectively address needs of disabled people. Others, such as Medicaid, did not.

American caregiving and American families have changed greatly since Pearl Buck and others described their predicament half a century ago. Some of the same basic challenges remain acute: support and comfort for caregivers, practical help and accurate information suited to families' specific situations, forming a reliable long-term arrangement that will work after the primary caregiver herself is gone. Public fear and stigma have abated, though families still confront private pain and loss that comes from significant intellectual disability. Community services are more extensive, though the relentlessness of the caregiving task remains daunting.

Policymakers still lack strong administrative structures to track family circumstances or to promote policy learning. For example, most disabled persons who reside with older caregivers are receiving Social Security or SSI payments administered by these same caregivers under representative payee arrangements. No systematic policy seeks to address this challenge.[57]

The dominant frame of compassion may even aggravate systemic weaknesses. Cancer patients and the chronically unemployed, like intellectually disabled citizens, require compassionate care. Yet in these arenas, compassion is understood as only part of an effective public response. Compassion must be disciplined by pertinent research and program evaluation, channeled through effective interventions.

Intellectual disability services are insulated from efforts to promote management innovation, evidence-based practice, and pay-for-performance that have improved other public health and medical care systems, notably the Veteran's Administration.[58] Agencies are provided funds sufficient to provide custodial care. They are expected to keep clients clean and safe, where possible to accommodate families' logistical needs. Agencies accomplish this mission though low labor costs with a low-skill workforce, with accompanying problems of morale and frequent turnover.[59] Within community-based settings, average hourly staff pay is $8.68.[60]

Policymakers struggle to provide families with the information needed to make wise choices within a decentralized network of community services. Few caregivers can accurately assess whether a daughter or brother receives the right mix of services. Many persons with intellectual disability experience complex co-morbidities. Many are treated by physicians and social service professionals who have limited experience in addressing these concerns.

Sixty years ago, caregiving was a private tragedy, in which parents cared for cognitively disabled children as best they could, for as long as they could. These burdens have not been lifted, but reducing them is now recognized as a proper task of public policy. This deserves celebration but does not guarantee success. Once again, our narrowly targeted altruism and our fragmented public sector conspire against our best efforts to help.

School of Social Service Administration
University of Chicago

Notes

1. James W. Trent, *Inventing the Feeble Mind: A History of Mental Retardation in the United States* (Berkeley and Los Angeles, 1994). Trent provides the essential starting reference in the social history of intellectual disability. His narrative provides a starting point for this article, though Trent does not focus strongly on income support or public aid policies considered here.

2. Paul J. Castellani, *From Snake Pits to Cash Cows* (Albany, N.Y., 2005).

3. The citation to *Pilgrim's Progress* is given by Trent, *Inventing the Feeble Mind*. Richard Herrnstein and Charles Murray, *The Bell Curve* (New York, 1994).

4. Janice A. Brockley, "Rearing the Child Who Never Grew," in *Mental Retardation in America*, ed. Steven Noll and James W. Trent (New York, 2004); Michael Bérubé, *Life as We Know It: A Father, a Family, and an Exceptional Child* (New York, 1996).

5. Hugh Heclo, "The Political Foundations of Anti-Poverty Policy," in *Fighting Poverty: What Works and What Doesn't*, ed. Sheldon Danziger and Donald Weinberg (Cambridge, Mass., 1986). R. Kent Weaver, *Ending Welfare as We Know It* (Washington, D.C., 2000).

6. Trent, *Inventing the Feebl Mind.*

7. Philip Reilly, *The Surgical Solution: A History of Involuntary Sterilization in the United States* (Baltimore, 2001).

8. Kathleen W. Jones, "Education for Children with Mental Retardation," in *Mental Retardation in America*, ed. Steven Noll and James W. Trent.

9. This story is best told by David J. Rothman and Sheila M Rothman, *The Willowbrook Wars* (New York, 1984).

10. Channing Richardson, "A Hundred-thousand Defectives," *Christian Century* 23 (January 1946): 110–11. I encountered this account in Trent, *Inventing the Feeble Mind.*

11. David A. Felicetti, *Mental Health and Retardation Politics* (New York, 1975). Conditions such as schizophrenia initially garnered the lion's share of NIMH expenditures.

12. Robert Segal, *The National Association for Retarded Citizens.* Arc 1974 [cited 29 May 2006]. Available from http://www.thearc.org/history/segal.htm.

13. David Braddock, Mary C. Rizzolo, Richard Hemp, and Susan L. Parish, "Public Spending for Developmental Disabilities in the United States," in *Costs and Outcomes of Community Services for People with Developmental Disabilities,* ed. R. Stancliffe and K. Lakin (Baltimore, 2005).

14. National Research Council, "Mental Retardation: Determining Eligibility for Social Security Benefits" (Washington, D.C., 2002).

15. None of the first-person caregiving accounts referenced in this article discuss public income-support programs for intellectually disabled persons, a telling reflection of the class position of those writing these accounts.

16. Pear S. Buck, *The Child Who Never Grew.* 2d ed. (Bethesda, Md., 1992).

17. Dale Evans Rogers, *Angel Unaware* (Westwood, N.J., 1953). See also Joseph Frank, *My Son's Story* (New York, 1952), and Charlotte D. Tucker, *Betty Lee* (New York, 1954). For contrast, see Bérubé, *Life as We Know It.*

18. Janice A. Brockley, "Rearing the Child Who Never Grew."

19. Other examples include Frank, *My Son's Story* and Tucker, *Betty Lee.*

20. Brockley, "Rearing the Child Who Never Grew."

21. Carol Levine, *Always on Call: When Illness Turns Families into Caregivers* (New York, 2000); Veronica P. Pollack and Harold A Pollack, "Bringing Vincent Home," *Health Affairs* 25, no. 1 (2006): 231–36.

22. This citation was drawn from Susan Rose-Ackerman, "Mental Retardation and Society: The Ethics and Politics of Normalization," *Ethics* 93, no. 1 (1982): 81–101.

23. On such anxieties, see Reilly, *Surgical Solution.*

24. David Strauss and Richard K. Eyman, "Mortality of People with Mental Retardation in California with and without Down Syndrome, 1986–1991," *American Journal of Mental Retardation* 100, no. 6 (1991): 643–53.

25. Kathleen Castles, "Nice Average Parents," in *Mental Retardation in America,* ed. Steven Noll and James W. Trent; Jones, "Education for Children with Mental Retardation."

26. Brockley, "Rearing the Child Who Never Grew."

27. Trent, *Inventing the Feeble Mind*; Segal, *The National Association for Retarded Citizens.*

28. Segal, *The National Association for Retarded Citizens.*

29. Cited in ibid.

30. Edward D. Berkowitz, *Disabled Policy* (Cambridge, 1987).

31. Humphrey Taylor, *Thirteenth Anniversary of the Americans with Disabilities Act (ADA).* Harris Interactive 2003 [cited July 12 2006]. Available from http://www.harrisinteractive.com/harris_poll/printerfriend/index.asp?PID=390.

32. David Neal and David L. Kirp, "The Allure of Legalization Reconsidered: The Case of Special Education, *Law and Contemporary Problems* 48, no. 1 (1985): 63–87.

33. Bowen Garrett and Sherry Glied, "Does State AFDC Generosity Affect Child SSI Participation? *Journal of Policy Analysis and Management* 19, no. 2 (2000): 275–95. The classic analysis of legal strategies is R. Shep Melnick, *Between the Lines: Interpreting Welfare Rights* (Washington, D.C., 1994).

34. The *Wall Street Journal* features especially prominent coverage of intellectual disability. See, for example, Claire Ansberry, "Disabled People Find Group Homes Can Be Broken, Too; Patients Gain Independence, but Oversight Is Spotty; Challenges of monitoring," *Wall Street Journal,* 13 September 2005, 1. Amy D. Marcus, "Eli's Choice," *Wall Street Journal,* 31 December, 1.

35. US-DHHS, 2003 Annual Statistical Report on the Social Security Disability Insurance Program (Washington, D.C., 2004).

36. Braddock, *Costs and Outcomes of Community Services for People with Developmental Disabilities*.

37. David Braddock, Richard Hemp, Mary C. Rizzolo, Diane Coulter, Laura Haffer, and Micah Thompson, *The State of the States in Developmental Disabilities 2005* (Boulder, Colo., 2006).

38. Max A. Murray, "Needs of Parents of Mentally Retarded Children, *American Journal of Mental Deficiency* (May 1959).

39. Arc, *The Arc's Logo and Name Changes Throughout Its History* 2006 [cited May 29 2006]. Available from http://www.thearc.org/history/names.htm.

40. Marsha M Seltzer, Marty W Krauss, Jinkuk Hong, and Gael I. Orsmond, "Continuity or Discontinuity of Family Involvement Following Residential Transitions of Adults Who Have Mental Retardation," *Mental Retardation* 39, no. 3 (2001): 181–94.

41. Trent, *Inventing the Feeble Mind*; Tucker, *Betty Lee*; Buck, *The Child Who Never Grew*.

42. Jeffrey Zaslow, "The Graduates: What Happens After Young Disabled Adults Leave School," *Wall Street Journal*, 29 December 2005, A1.

43. Braddock, *The State of the States in Developmental Disabilities*.

44. Pollack and Pollack, "Bringing Vincent Home."

45. Joe Brian Soss, *Unwanted Claims: The Politics of Participation in the U.S. Welfare Wystem* (Ann Arbor, 2002).

46. Braddock, *The State of the States in Developmental Disabilities*.

47. This paragraph draws on Pollack and Pollack, "Bringing Vincent Home."

48. Theresa M. Varnet, *Special Needs Trust Ensures Support, Care* (Chicago, 1998).

49. Ansberry, "Disabled People Find Group Homes Can Be Broken, Too."

50. Avram Goldstein and Katherine Boo, "D.C. Vows Review of Deaths in Homes: Care of the Retarded to Face New Oversight," *Washington Post*, 6 December 1999, 1.

51. Melnick, *Between the Lines: Interpreting Welfare Rights*.

52. Ibid.; Neal and Kirp, "The Allure of Legalization Reconsidered."

53. Rothman and Rothman, *Willowbrook Wars*.

54. Theda Skocpol, *Protecting Soldiers and Mothers* (Cambridge, Mass., 1995), 527–28.

55. Melnick, *Between the Lines: Interpreting Welfare Rights*.

56. Ibid.

57. Such problems are rarely addressed in academic research. If one searches Medline for the terms "developmental disability" and "representative payee," one finds no article addressing intergenerational succession in caregiving.

58. See, for example, Ashish K. Jha, Jonathan B. Perlin, Kenneth W. Kizer, and R. Adams Dudley, "Effect of the Transformation of the Veterans Affairs Health Care System on the Quality of Care," *New England Journal of Medicine* 348, no. 22 (2003): 2218–27.

59. K. Charlie Lakin, Barbara Polister, and Robert W. Prouty, "Wages of Non-state Direct Support Professionals Lag Behind Those of Public Direct Support Professionals and the General Public," *Mental Retardation* 41, no. 2 (2003): 178–82.

60. Braddock, *The State of the States in Developmental Disabilities*.

BRETT L. WALKER

Sanemori's Revenge: Insects, Eco-System Accidents, and Policy Decisions in Japan's Environmental History

Normally we do not think of living organisms as machines or as relays in complex, tightly coupled technological systems. Nonetheless, in recent years this is precisely the manner in which many environmental histori-ans have come to approach the study of certain organisms and their natural or anthropogenic environments.[1] Over the millennia and across the globe, humans have so manipulated certain organisms that they have come to exist solely as parts of technological systems or industrialized chains of production and consumption. Technological artifacts are, of course, only nature refashioned: nonetheless, modern industrialized societies tend to view themselves as gradually distancing themselves from, replacing, or, in some instances, even killing nature with their advanced technologies and gadgetries, when actually they are only refashioning their inseparable relationship to it.[2]

For the purposes of this article, two assumptions are critical to seeing organisms as technologies or as parts of technological systems. The first is that humans are capable of shaping the evolution of other crea-tures on this planet—in some instances our species has even caused the creation of new species, or "speciation"[3]—and that meaningful evolution can occur over the course of years and not only eons. That is, as historian Edmund Russell, a major proponent of "evolutionary history," has argued, "Organisms have changed in historical time" due to intentional and unintentional human meddling with three keystone Darwinian factors: variation, inheritance, and selection. Russell continues that inves-tigating the manner in which human histories have shaped the evolution of other organisms allows us to "historicize organisms themselves," which carves out a new place for historians in generating knowledge about the current state of evolution and the natural world.[4] Historicizing organisms means that historians can trace the manner in which policy decisions, whether by silkworm cultivators, pesticide producers, or government extension agencies, have influenced the evolution of certain organisms.

The second assumption is this: if humans manipulate the evolution of certain organisms, then this manipulation, whether intentional or unintentional, resembles the manipulation of metals and electronic circuitries in machines or other conventional technologies or technological systems. Russell helps us navigate this tricky theoretical terrain as well. Strictly speaking, he explains, organisms are not conventional machines but rather are "biological artifacts shaped by humans to serve human ends." This represents a merger of technology and nature, not a separation or an instance of one killing the other. Take agriculture. As Russell explains, "No one has yet figured out how to transform sunlight, carbon dioxide, and a few nutrients into grain—except by subcontracting the job to plants. The same goes for meat production and animals."

Needless to say, industrialization is an important part of this process. As Russell points out, in the case of industrialized agriculture, "Biological development was roughly as important as mechanical innovation in boosting productivity." For farmers, that is, new hybrid grains and improved chicken breeds prove just as important in boosting production as do new threshers, combines, and mechanical feather removers. Today, farms resemble factories, and consumers, when perusing supermarket aisles, shop for carefully disassembled "legs and thighs" for their specific caloric demands.[5] More still, when we adopt "evolutionary history" as our analytical starting point, it allows us to think more co-evolutionarily as well.[6] We begin to see "not just how humans shape organisms, but how organisms shape humans."[7] Apparently, modern people, too, are products of their interaction with other organisms and, therefore, of their own co-evolutionary history.

Insects prove to be wonderful examples of organisms evolving as a result of human activities: insects such as bees and silkworms serve as biotechnologies; others develop hereditary resistances to certain pesticides. In other words, insects serve as technologies, but they also serve as targets of technologies, which causes them to evolve through developing resistances. Flying scale insects, nematode worms, and some ticks have reportedly developed resistances to such powerful toxins as buquinolate, thiabendazole, and HCH/dieldrin in only a matter of a few generations because their lifecycles are relatively short. Policy decisions play the following role: federal officials, such as those in the Agricultural Research Service (a division of the U.S. Department of Agriculture), devised strategies to use insecticides based on certain economic and political considerations related to their ties to the chemical industry and, consequently, people suffered debilitating health problems from toxic drift caused by overspraying.[8] Surely, one of the best examples of derelict public policy decisions related to insecticide use is the "fire ant wars," campaigns waged against an insect that, most serious entomologists agreed, posed little economic threat to agriculture, but nonetheless became the target of chlorinated hydrocarbon saturations that ravaged rural ecosystems and human health in the American South.[9] However, insects also developed hereditary resistances as a result of bad science and poor policy decisions. In Africa, some mosquitoes evolved in a manner that allowed them to avoid DDT sprayed in village huts; other mosquitoes, such as the tenacious *Culex pipiens*, can withstand normally lethal doses of organophosphate insecticides because it actually digests the poison.[10] In each instance, policy decisions, whether in the form of agricultural policies, public health strategies, or experimentation by pesticide producers, shaped the evolution of insects or caused human health problems as a result of ecosystem degradation.

That is to say, not just insects, but the rice paddies and other agricultural landscapes they inhabit need to be seen as technological "eco-systems." Modern rice paddies are not disorganized, unstructured landscapes, but rather are carefully parceled, highly organized segments of land, arranged in a systematic manner to increase yields and ease production. Simply, the modern farm is a factory: a complex ecological system or artificial ecosystem.[11] When sprayed, insecticides become part of insect bodies and alter their evolution through inducing resistances; but even more important, these toxins become a part of the rural ecosystems that insects inhabit, leading to systemic "normal accidents," as Charles Perrow has called them, that result from the complex, tightly coupled nature of modern agriculture. The "eco-system accident," explains Perrow, is the "interaction of systems that were thought to be independent but are not because of the larger ecology." One example of an unforeseen consequence of spraying insecticides on paddies is the biomagnification of toxins in the living tissue of organisms.[12] Perrow writes, "Eco-system accidents illustrate the tight coupling between human-made systems and natural systems. There are few or no deliberate buffers inserted between the two systems because the designers never expected them to be connected."[13]

But they are seamlessly connected. When it comes to agriculture, modern people are as much a part of the tightly coupled, complex ecosystem as everything else and, hence, prove vulnerable to system accidents in the form of toxic pollution. That is this article's main point: many environmental problems, from poisoned landscapes to disfigured fetuses, can be seen as the products of system accidents caused by policy decisions that resonate throughout hybridized environments, but only if we trace these toxins from the government and corporate organizations that sponsor and produce them, through the social networks that disseminate them, into the ecosystems that disperse them, to the human and nonhuman bodies that absorb them and, ultimately, sicken and die from them.[14] Every time we put a morsel of food into our mouths, from shiny sushi rice to crispy fried chicken, we reify our organic interface with policy decisions made in corporations, agribusiness farms, and government ministries.

This article examines six case studies of how decisions made in chemical companies, government ministries, and religious organizations led to the "historical evolution" of certain organisms or to deadly "ecosystem accidents," ones that ruined the health of Japanese bodies. Our first case study is an industrial organism that served Japanese fashion rather than caloric needs: silkworms, the world's only completely domesticated insect.

Silkworms

Silkworms (*Bombyx mori*) serve as organisms that humans have, over centuries, transformed into purely industrial technologies: their survival remains utterly dependent on human beings. Today, tucked away in institutions such as "stock centers" at a handful of major East Asian universities are hundreds of Mendelian mutations of the silkworm, most of them spontaneously discovered by cultivators and then preserved; other mutations scientists induced through irradiation techniques and chemical mutagenesis. Many of these mutations represent "improved strains," or silkworms that exhibit economically desirable qualities such as rapid growth rate, cocoon size, silk filament quality, and disease resistances. Silkworms from southwestern China, for example, prove desirable because of their hereditary resistance to toxic fluoride levels in mulberry leaves, an environmental condition caused by the brick industry in that region. In effect, this is historical evolution in action: the brick industry produced environmental toxins that, over historical time, induced selection among silkworms, leading to evolutionary mutations among the organisms. This beneficial "gene," in turn, has been isolated and preserved by certain institutions for future breeding purposes.[15]

In the case of Japan, stylistic idiosyncrasies, ones that have evolved since Heian-period (794–1185) female courtiers wore some eighty pounds of silk clothing carefully chosen to match learned cultural sensibilities, influenced the evolution of silkworms as well, because only certain bugs produced the desirable high-quality filament.[16] Today, functional genomics has allowed institutions to engineer silkworms that produce such specialized silks, as well as recombinant proteins made in the silk glands with beneficial pharmacological qualities. Indeed, within certain institutions, Japanese scientists have accumulated entire databases that hold silkworm DNA, from where they distribute clones internationally for commercial and scientific use.[17] Because no wild silkworms exist (their closest relative is *Bombyx mandarina*), they represent one of the oldest examples of historical evolution and organisms being used as industrial technologies. Certainly in Japan, silkworms have depended on their doting human providers, mostly women, for millennia.

Silkworms have long been in Japan, as evidenced by eighth-century creation mythologies. During one divine encounter narrated in the *Kojiki* (Record of Ancient Matters; 712), the intrepid, but also quite hungry, deity Susano'o kills the food deity, Ogetsuhime, because he thought she sought to pollute him by pulling various foodstuffs out of her nose, mouth, and anus. Evidencing the importance of silkworms in Japan's ancient mythologies and economies, from Ogetsuhime's divine corpse grew the vital grains—the foodstuffs on which Japanese have endured for centuries—and also silkworms.[18] The myth explains, "In the corpse of the slain deity there grew [various] things: in her head there grew silkworms; in her two eyes there grew rice seeds; in her two ears there grew millet; in her nose there grew red beans; in her genitals there grew wheat; and in her rectum there grew soy beans."[19] In others words, Japanese wove silkworm cultivation into the deepest fibers of their cultural fabric; and the caterpillar's incremental domestication paralleled the domestication of Japan's earliest food crops.

Preindustrial rural households tended their silkworm nurseries with the same sort of care that they did their rice, millet, bean, wheat, and soybean fields. For the past two centuries, when rural households purchased silkworm eggs, often they exchanged no money and the agent simply deducted his proceeds when the worms had spun their precious silk cocoons. Until they hatched, often as many as twenty thousand of these eggs laid spread out on wooden trays; once hatched, farmers carefully brushed the squirming larvae onto rearing trays using a soft feather so as to not crush their tiny bodies. Farmers covered the rearing trays in wet rice husks to provide the necessary humidity and then spread out a layer of chopped white mulberry (*Morus alba*) leaves for the silkworms to munch on. Often families sacrificed their sleeping space to provide comfortable accommodations for these bugs.

For about three days the larvae devoured carefully cut mulberry leaves; on the fourth day they hibernated. But then they shed and were reborn, with gauzy skin and bright stripes down their bodies. Such metamorphic qualities—their biological ability to change into completely different creatures—did not go unnoticed by the Japanese and insects became potent symbols of Buddhist notions of transmigration: when the soul, in the endless cycle of birth and rebirth, travels to the next life after this one. Eighth-century mythmakers marveled in the *Kojiki* at the metamorphic quality of silkworms as well. "Among the insects raised by Nurinomi," a fourth-century migrant to Japan, "there is a strange variety of insect that changes three ways; first it becomes a crawling worm, then again it becomes a cocoon, then once again it becomes a flying bird."[20] As with the East Asian writing system (called *kanji* in Japanese) and other technologies and institutions, sericulture was perfected by migrants who came to Japan on well-trodden migration circuits between the fourth and eighth centuries, mainly from the Korean peninsula.

In nurseries, by the fifth or sixth day, silkworms grew to the point where cultivators needed to carefully spread them out on even more trays, with an ever-ready supply of fresh mulberry leaves. Silkworms grew at a tremendous rate and, by the time they started spinning their silk, they weighed some ten thousand times their weight as larvae. The silkworms ate and molted and ate and molted some four times in all, until, after their final metamorphosis, they prepared to spin their cocoons by eating steadily for six days straight. By this time, the silkworms measured about one to two inches in length, walked dexterously for having eight sets of legs: three sets of jointed legs, with a sole claw at the tip, and five sets of fleshy leglike protrusions with hooks for climbing and clinging. They also sported a lavishly decorative short "anal horn" on their backs. When in the larval stage, silkworms preferred the delicate shoots from the tops of the mulberry, but later, when adults, they ate everything even remotely mulberry: the some twenty thousand larvae cultivated by one rural household consumed a total of thirteen hundred pounds of leaves.

Farmers set aside thousands of acres for growing mulberry to feed hungry caterpillars, often when there was barely enough land to grow grain to feed the people of their villages. In the eighteenth century, some of the best agricultural lands around Japan's major cities—in the Kanto Plain around Tokyo and the Kinai and Kansai areas around Kyoto and Osaka—farmers replanted with mulberry and land for raising vital human food crops, such as soybean, sprang up in more distant areas in the northeast and elsewhere. The market demand for foodstuffs to feed hungry urban populations forced a monoculture regimen on distant areas such as Hachinohe in the far northeast, setting the region up for devastating famine when soybean crops failed because of weather and, in one bizarre instance, exploding populations of hungry wild boar.[21] All this so that mulberry trees could be cultivated to feed more and more hungry bugs. This is the essence of co-evolution: humans sacrificing their own precious farming lands to feed hungry bugs on whom they depend economically. Indeed, with their tiny heads, silkworms must have nodded with satisfaction as Japanese farmers eliminated rice and soybean croplands to make room for more mulberries and refashioned lending patterns, risked awful debt, kept children at home, and sacrificed their already squalid living space just to nurture them.

When silkworms began spinning, families designed special frames for them to hang from. Timing was critical at this stage, because the worms had to be ready to spin their cocoon; they simply soiled the cocoons of others if they were not and this ruined the quality of the silk. Over the next several days, the family eagerly watched as the worms went to work on their beautiful translucent cocoons made from thread excreted from special glands: a piece of evolutionary hardware that has allowed these creatures to be treated with such care. Once they completed the cocoon, they molted one final time, and eager farmers raced the cocoons to silk agents to collect their earnings. Farmers boiled poor-quality cocoons to make silk thread for their own clothing; some ate the plump, protein-rich insects or fed them to fish in communally tended ponds. Little was left to waste in preindustrial Japan. Later, in the period just before the Pacific War (1937–45), silk agents paid between one and two hundred yen for these cocoons. (One cocoon could produce more than fifteen hundred feet of valuable silk thread.) Obviously, when entire colonies of silkworms perished, it financially wiped out these already deeply impoverished rural households, who famously produced no less than 70 percent of Meiji tax revenues through absolutely crushing land taxes.[22] Rural families shouldered financially Japan's industrialization; they did so environmentally, too.

The silkworm provides an excellent example of an industrialized organism whose life has been shaped by policy decisions made by cultivators and rural lending institutions, ones that are then transferred through economic systems, social networks, and rural ecosystems. Silkworms symbolize our intentional and unintentional meddling: creatures that evolved according to the needs of our economic, cultural, social, and ecological systems. Think of it this way: the Japanese desired certain silk fabric from certain kinds of caterpillars because of traditional cultural sensibilities; the Japanese bought silkworms in the manner they did because of the development of rural financial institutions; and the Japanese, particularly the smaller, dexterous hands of women, raised silkworms in homes because patrilocal Confucian kinship patterns had sequestered them there.[23]

Insects, Buddhism, and Japanese B Encephalitis

Our second case study examines the manner in which cultural sensibilities inherent in Buddhism and biogeographical ones inherent in Japan's nineteenth-century decision to adopt industrial agriculture led to the creation of ideal habitat for certain mosquitoes that carried neurological diseases that threatened human health. Biologically, silkworms underwent three distinct transformations on their way to their final destination of becoming a moth. For this evolutionary talent, the Japanese associated such insects as silkworms, butterflies, cicadas, and mosquitoes with metamorphic qualities likened to the cyclical nature of human existence according to Buddhist cosmologies. Insects such as silkworms and cicadas started out as eggs, they hatched and became hungry larvae, they matured to even hungrier pupa, and, in their final transcendence, they sprouted wings. For this reason, Japanese literary classics are littered with insect references, usually alluding to the sadness or the impermanence of this transient world.[24]

In the nineteenth century, Lafcadio Hearn (1850–1904), an American living in Japan, wrote lengthy meditations on insects and Buddhist notions of impermanence. Hearn lived in Japan in the metamorphic Meiji years (1868–1912), when Japan itself shed its skin, and he lamented the cruel destruction of an older Japan in favor of the new industrial order. Similar to the silkworms and cicadas he observed, Hearn too underwent a metamorphosis while living in Japan when he adopted the Japanese name Koizumi Yakumo and, in his own mind, sprouted wings and became in many respects "Japanese."[25] When writing about butterflies, Hearn retrieved ancient Japanese and Chinese myths that the souls of the deceased wandered this world in the form of butterflies, sometimes eavesdropping on former lovers. According to another story, butterflies descended on the ancient capital of Kyoto by the thousands in the tenth century and, in doing so, portended the countless men to be killed and resurrected as insects during the rebellion of Taira no Masakado (d. 940).

But Hearn also tied the fate of mosquitoes to the fate of the older Japan he cherished. The mosquitoes that infested his Tokyo neighborhood and stung him originated in a deeply spiritual place, in a nearby cemetery, where, at the foot of ancient, moss-covered Buddhist tombs, worshipers placed water in *mizutame* (cisterns) so that the souls of the dead, when reborn and preparing for their otherworldly journey, could satisfy their insatiable thirst. But his neighborhood cemetery was an old one, and the standing water in the tens of thousands of cisterns and flower receptacles proved excellent breeding habitat for mosquitoes—under Meiji Japan's hygienic regimen, a health risk. The mosquitoes that so pestered Hearn and other Tokyoites rose "by the millions from the water of the dead," he wrote. He speculated, referring to Buddhism's six realms of existence, that "some of them may be reincarnations of those very dead, condemned by the error of former lives" to wander the earth as blood-suckers. He marveled that "some wicked human soul had been compressed into that wailing speck of a body."[26]

Here Buddhist orthodoxies intersected with ecological systems, and the cisterns and vessels left at the cemetery provided water for transmigrating souls as well as prime breeding habitat for mosquitoes: religious practices and cultural sensibilities interfaced with ecological ones and caused an urban health crisis. That is, had it not been for the religious demand for cisterns, the cascading and unforeseen "ecosystem accidents" that resulted from these cemeteries would not have occurred. Indeed, these swarms of Japanese insects represented a serious threat in the eyes of a Meiji government increasingly concerned with national discipline through the health and hygiene of Japan's citizenry. Some of the mosquitoes (*Culex tritaeniorhynchus*) born in these Buddhist cisterns carried the "arbovirus" (arthropod-borne virus) that causes Japanese B encephalitis. Normally, these mosquitoes live and breed in the marshy paddy lands of rural Japan, but standing water in cities attracts them as well. One reason the mosquito-borne disease thrived in rural areas, but later came to the outskirts of cities, was because this peculiar virus spends part of its lifecycle in the bodies of pigs, who serve as an "amplifying host." With the advent of modern agriculture (there had been little animal husbandry in preindustrial Japan), vast numbers of pigs came to live near human populations.[27] Between 1926 and 1938, about the same time that several high-profile Japanese B encephalitis outbreaks occurred, Japan witnessed nearly a 100 percent increase in its pig population, from 504,758 to 997,980. Although small rural cultivators raised most of these pigs, some large-scale producers, according to later U.S. occupation documents, were "located on the outskirts of the large cities," where the animals had easy access to garbage for feed.[28] Obviously, the decision to place large concentrations of pigs near cities (and their accompanying cemeteries with mosquitoes and, nearby, human populations) set Japan up for "eco-system accidents" in the form of Japanese B encephalitis epidemics.

Mosquitoes sucked the blood of these pigs and transported the blood-borne, amplified virus to nearby human hosts. Most people do not develop severe symptoms of Japanese B encephalitis, but when they do, the disease can be devastating, causing death or brain damage and paralysis. In 1924, some 6,000 reported cases of encephalitis left 3,800 people dead in Tokyo alone; that same year, the disease also occurred in Kagawa District of Kyushu, where 60 percent of those who contracted the affliction—some 3,500 souls—died of fever and brain swelling. Japanese B encephalitis was also one of a host of afflictions that plagued Japan immediately after the surrender to the Allies in 1945.[29]

A ghoulish aside to our story of encephalitis is Ishii Shiro (1892–1959), the eccentric young Japanese biologist who invented the filtration device that proved instrumental in isolating and identifying the virus. His career later proved a sinister one, as he applied his scientific expertise in water impurities, filtration, arboviruses, and insects to develop Japan's biological weapons program in China.[30] Although outside the scope of this article, Ishii oversaw a biological weapons program in China during the Pacific War, which, among other horrific enterprises, raised bubonic-plague-carrying fleas in nurseries (much in the manner that villagers had raised silkworms), packed them in bombs in swabs of cotton, and then released them over Chinese cities such as Ningbo (27 October 1940) and Changde (11 April 1942).[31] The Japanese killed thousands of Chinese civilians with this military biotechnology. This policy linkage between killing anthropoids and arthropods is not surprising, however. The same European and American companies that developed chemicals and aerial dispersal technologies to kill bugs easily transferred them to human battlefields and visa versa during times of war.[32]

To summarize, the manner in which Japanese viewed the transmigration of the soul, modern agricultural, and their "vermin" Chinese neighbors in times of war, led to epidemiological outbursts of Japanese B encephalitis and epidemics of bubonic plague. Policy decisions underwritten by religion, agriculture, and ethno-nationalism interfaced to threaten the health of human bodies at home and abroad. But explanations of the transmigration of the soul also shaped how rural Japanese explained the outbreak of famine.[33] One of the best-known historical examples of insects causing severe crop damage and famine in Japan—insects harming Japan's earliest hybrid agricultural systems—is the Kyoho famine. In the following examination, Buddhist attitudes toward the transmigration of the soul shaped Japan's initial foray into "economic entomology," because tackling the threat caused by agricultural pests meant placating the former humans whose souls inhabit the tiny, buzzing bodies of insects such as plant hoppers and locusts.

Early Modern Japanese Famines and Insecticides

The Kyoho famine of 1732–one of Japan's three "great famines" of the early modern period (1600–1868)—was partially caused by insects and, after its outbreak, ravaged central and western Japan, particularly the islands of Kyushu and Shikoku. *Unka*, or plant hoppers of various subspecies, represented the principal troublemakers during the 1732 famine: farmers reported, in the beginning of the sixth month of the lunar calendar, massive emergences of one species of rice plant hoppers (*Sogatella furcifera*) and, about two weeks later, a second wave of a different species (*Nilaparvata lugens*). To this day, these delphacid insects represent serious threats to rice crops throughout Asia, though in temperate climates, such as those in Korea and Japan, the hoppers do not survive the winter. They therefore travel to these countries on seasonal winds from southeastern China, coordinating their arrival with the transplanting of lush, green rice crops in spring and early summer.[34] In 1732, hoppers coordinated their arrival perfectly, and Kyushu farmers reported widespread crop damage as a result of these two waves of insect invaders.

In other locations, such as in Komatsu domain, in Iyo province on Shikoku Island, farmers reported insect damage in the form of *mushigui*, a reference to hoppers infesting rice stalks and sucking these plants dry of their life-giving juices until they simply withered, turned brown, and died. So many hoppers swam on the surface of the paddies that the water turned "the color of soy sauce." During the day, the hoppers stayed on the rice stalks, contently sucking the juices; at night, however, when farmers inspected the crops with pine torches, they saw that the insects had moved to the heads of the plants, where they ate the precious grain itself. Despite prayers offered at temples and shrines to disperse the insects, crops turned brown, withered, and died; farmers watched helplessly as insects less than an inch long unceremoniously consumed bushel upon bushel of the gold standard of Japan's early modern political economy.[35]

Not only cultivators in Komatsu, but those in Hiroshima domain experienced hopper infestations as well: they peaked around the sixteenth or seventeenth day of the seventh month of the lunar calendar. Farmers described the hoppers as having risen up from the "earth's vapors" to resemble giant plumes of noxious smoke hovering over the crops. Farmers also noticed, however, that during the first ten days of the eighth month, when temperatures dropped, the hoppers died off, because they coped poorly with Japan's temperate climate. Farmers in the five home provinces around the ancient capital of Kyoto—the Kinai region—similarly reported infestations of hoppers so large (probably a third wave of the leaf hopper *Cicadula sexnotata*) that they resembled the "golden coin beetle," a pesky insect known in the United States as the "Japanese beetle." Farmers explained that the hoppers sported an exoskeleton that resembled protective armor, that they flew, and that in one night a swarm of them ate the equivalent of literally tens of thousands of bushels of rice. In the Kinai, farmers compared the hoppers to the "golden coin beetle," but in the western provinces they referred to the pest as Sanemori. Just as Lafcadio Hearn had ruminated on the transmigratory lives of mosquitoes in a nearby cemetery, farmers in Japan's western provinces believed that the insects were actually the spirit of the vengeful general Saito Betto Sanemori (1111-83), who, in the twelfth-century, had died in the fields of Shinohara of Kaga Province at the hands of rival Tetsuka Mitsumori.[36] Farmers believed that Sanemori continued to hold a grudge against the farmers of western Japan and so he came back in the bodies of plant hoppers to ruin their rice crops: this was the principle behind their Buddhist-inspired entomology. It also shaped how early modern rural entomologists sought to eliminate the threat caused by these pests.

To frighten off the spirit of Sanemori, farmers from the western provinces fashioned scarecrows from straw, which they strategically placed along coastal shorelines or on the borders of their villages and rice paddies. When Sanemori (now better armored than in the twelfth century) ignored these straw men, farmers employed what they referred to as the "oil extermination" technique by pouring rapeseed or whale oil on the water of their paddies in order to suffocate hoppers that fell into the water. This "oil extermination" method represents one of the first uses of insecticides in Japan. Rural lore explains that resourceful farmers invented the "oil extermination" technique in Chikuzen province, on Kyushu Island, in 1670, but later improved on the technique by lighting it and burning the insects alive. A treatise on "insect control" by Okura Nagatsune (1766-1860) contains illustrations that depict farmers burning hoppers with oil and pine torches. Apparently the technique was discovered when, one night, a man named Yahiro, while lighting temple lamps, noticed that hoppers flew into the lit oil and died, and so desperate farmers replicated the technique on a larger scale. In Fukuoka domain, also in Chikuzen, farmers called the hopper infestations a "vision of Michizane's Dazaifu spirit," a reference to legendary classical scholar and statesman Sugawara no Michizane (845–903). On being exiled by political rivals to Dazaifu, capital of the western provinces (in present-day Fukuoka prefecture), Michizane died in disgrace, but, shortly after his death, his rivals in Kyoto began dying too, and so north of Kyoto a shrine was erected in honor of "Tenman Tenjin," his posthumous, deified name. His spirit remains associated with rigorous scholarship and continues to grace smart young Japanese entrance-examination-takers to this day. Farmers in Fukuoka, close to Michizane's grave, no doubt assumed that he had taken the form of plant hoppers, much as Sanemori had in Kaga province.[37]

Okura Nagatsune's "insect control" treatise, entitled *Jokoroku*, serves as a fascinating example of the methods used by rural cultivators to protect their crops and exterminate plant hoppers and locusts. He began the treatise by observing that, in times of unseasonable weather, plant hoppers and other rice-eating insects (*unka*) appear on rice crops and, after severely damaging them, famine often results. Famine, he insisted, represented the "number one affliction of the realm." In retrospect, he was probably right. He continued that "farmers must learn the methods of preventing [damage caused by] plant hoppers" if the realm-wide scourge of famine was to be eliminated. Okura's principal example of the dangers of insects and famine was the Kyoho episode; but he recalled the intense hardships of the Tenmei famine as well, specifically the unseasonable weather of 1783 and 1787, when he was a young child growing up in Hitashi in Bungo province (present-day Oita prefecture). So he knew from personal experiences the dangers of insects and famine and sought to prevent it through the use of insecticides.[38]

During the Kyoho famine, farmers tried these and other methods of insect control. Fukuoka farmers applied nearly one gallon of "fish oil" per acre to rid their paddies of the angry Michizane: Japanese refashioned fish and whales into technologies of insect eradication. The technique developed in Fukuoka quickly spread throughout the provinces of western Japan, as in Matsuyama domain, in Iyo province, farmers reportedly tried the technique in their paddies as well. But fish and whale oil proved expensive and beyond the economic means of most farmers; and the fact that the policy of domain lords, and even the Tokugawa shogun, was to order prayers at various temples, though magnanimous indeed, probably did little to stem the hopper tide. The shogun also had associated insects with disgruntled ghosts, and, in what we might see as an official Buddhist-inspired policy response, ordered prayers at Japan's most sacred sites, including such institutions as the Ise Shrine, the Grand Shrine at Izumo, Buzen Usa, Hitachi Kashima, Katori, Iwashi Mizuhachiman-gu, the Nikko mausoleum, the Enryakuji Temple at Mount Hiei, and Gojiin. When domain lords formally reported the damage done to crops, the shogun generously reduced their *mononari*, or yearly rice tribute, and even offered loans to the most devastated areas.[39]

Sadly, the cool temperatures in the eighth month that stemmed the tied of hungry plant hoppers also successfully killed off what remained of western Japan's rice crops. The combined damage from insects and unseasonable weather hit Matsuyama domain particularly hard, destroying most of its harvest. There, farmers desperately experimented with whale oil to kill insects, but the technique did little good and in 1732 the lord reported that 3,489 people had died of starvation, along with 1,694 oxen and 1,403 horses.[40] The Kyoho famine became known as one of early modern Japan's "three great famines," the others being the Tenmei and the Tenpo famines.[41] What makes it important is that, in the midst of the deadly crisis, Japan's earliest economic entomologists experimented with a variety of oils and techniques to rid crops of hungry plant hoppers, experiences that rural cultivators and their children's children carried with them into the modern age of agricultural science.

To review, policy decisions made by Japanese farmers or officials in the Tokugawa shogunate designed to tackle the deadly Kyoho famine—setting up scarecrows on the coastline, conjuring spells, worshiping at temples and shrines, anthropomorphizing insects with the transmigrating spirits of past statesmen, and relying on whale oil as an insecticide—expose how Buddhist sentiments, early agrarian technologies, and the Tokugawa government (and its reliance on the *kokudaka* system) directly shaped famine, the pathology of disease, and the nature of premature mortality in Japan. Here cosmological and agronomic systems intersected seamlessly with entomological ones: an example of the manner in which human-designed religious orthodoxies, government decisions, and technologies manifest themselves in the natural world.

Meiji Insecticides

Plant hoppers, locust, scale insects, and other insect pests proved no less dangerous under the Meiji government (1868–1912) than they had under the Tokugawa shoguns. But Meiji modernizers felt more pressure than ever to increase agricultural yields on croplands because, with industrialization, more people transferred from rural areas to newly constructed urban factories to work as laborers. So, in essence, Japan's working lands needed to feed and thereby fuel a growing industrial population with fewer people actually cultivating them.[42] For this reason, fertilizers and insecticides proved invaluable to Japan's modernization designs: in effect, farmers boosted yields with chemical fertilizers and, through increased use of insecticides, hoped to share fewer of their painstakingly produced calories with always-hungry six-legged competitors.

Early modern farmers processed whale blubber and rapeseeds and turned them into agents of insect control; Meiji Japanese sought other remedies to eradicate pests, remedies more chemical in nature. They deployed chemicals because the manner in which Japanese viewed agriculture and entomology changed: in the modern scientific order, casting spells, offering official prayers at shrines and temples, and setting up scarecrows smacked of a superstitious past. Chemicals, by contrast, represented the promise of Euro-American science, a new form of "magic," much as Buddhism has been centuries earlier, one rooted in economic entomology and advanced chemistry, not theories regarding the transmigration of Sanemori's bitter soul.

What set the Meiji approach apart was less a reliance on rural folk remedies and more an obsession with European and American science: the obsession with science translated into an early experimentation with simple chemical means of killing insects in the context of a more industrialized agricultural regimen.[43] And nowhere in nineteenth-century Japan was modern, industrialized agriculture more coveted than on the newly acquired island of Hokkaido, where the Kaitakushi (Hokkaido Development Agency) hired foreign experts from the United States and elsewhere to assist in the creation of modern agriculture on that island.[44] And, typical of nineteenth-century agricultural modernization in Japan, the United States, with its network of land-grant colleges, extension agencies, experiment stations, and state and federal development offices, provided Meiji policymakers with model institutions.

As early as the 1840s, U.S. economic entomologists had begun pushing for greater relevancy in the agricultural sciences. That is, they no longer wanted to be seen as quirky men with thick glasses, whose homes were cluttered with case upon case of needle-impaled insect specimens; they wanted to contribute to practical science, and they did so by conjuring up a war against insects in America's working lands. But there was a degree of reality to the war against insects: increasing urbanization had demanded more mono-crop agriculture to feed people, which made crops more susceptible to insect damage. In 1854, the U.S. government hired a lone entomologist to travel the country cataloging and collecting information on noxious insects; by 1868, the same year as the Meiji Restoration, some states followed suite and hired entomologists as well. At this early juncture, among the insecticides sprayed on crops throughout the United States in the nineteenth century was "Buhach" (the American proprietary name for pyrethrum powder), "Paris green" (a copper ace-toarsenate), "London purple" (basically calcium arsenate), "lead arsenate," and "Bordeaux mixture" (to be discussed below). Signs of trouble related to the use of such insecticides appeared early on, however. In 1891, for example, a public-health scare related to poisoned grapes and "Bordeaux mixture" rocked New York City; later, public health officials debated the degree to which arsenic, which cultivators sprayed liberally on fruit crops, caused chronic health problems among consumers. That is, the use of arsenic as an insecticide forced the medical community to grapple with the long-term chronic health consequences of arsenic poisoning.[45]

Drawing on the U.S. experience, Hokkaido's working lands became nothing less than laboratories—literally, experiment stations—where the Kaitakushi tested newly imported agriculture technologies, including chemical insecticides. One of these technologies was an inorganic carbon-sulfur compound used to combat scale insects in orchards as well as rusting disease on wheat crops in 1874. The compound "lime sulfur," as farmers commonly called it, proved effective against wheat crop and apple orchard diseases, such as fungal head blight (Gibberella zeae), wheat leaf rust (Puccinia triticina), and powdery mildew (Podosphaera leucotricha), as well as insects such as red mites (Metatetranychus citri) and arrowhead scales (Unaspis yanonensis). In 1881, moreover, Meiji modernizers began import-ing "pyrethrum powder" from England (made from chrysanthemums); four years later, they imported seeds for insect-repelling chrysanthemums from the United States and, once in Japan, farmers cultivated the plants throughout the country. The plants proved so successful that by 1898, Japan, with the support of the Meiji government, became an exporter of dried chrysanthemum flowers to the United States. Simultaneously, Japanese scientists experimented with a variety of chrysanthemum-based chemical insecticides, including mosquito incense. In 1901, Japanese agronomists developed a "chrysanthemum-petroleum emulsion" that farmers used as an insecticide throughout the country. More important, Japanese scientists participated in the development of "pyrethroid," a synthetic version of the naturally occurring "pyrethrum." This chemical proved to be one of the four big insecticides of its day.[46]

In 1897, Japanese agricultural organizations, such as the Japanese Association for the Prevention of Plant Disease (Nihon Shokubutsu Boeki

Kyokai) and the Japanese Association for Research into Regulated Chemicals (Nihon Shokubutsu Chosetsuzai Kenkyu Kyokai), also experimented with "Bordeaux mixture" at experiment grape vineyards in Japan. "Bordeaux mixture," developed by Pierre-Marie-Alexis Millardet (1838–1902) in the 1860s, is a fungicide and bactericide made from copper sulfate and hydrated lime. Other simple chemical compound insecticides and bactericides experimented with included hydrocyanic gas fumigants, Horumarin soil disinfectants, and arsenic acid; naturally occurring insecticides included sulfuric acid, nicotine, and Rotenone.

At experiment stations and elsewhere, Meiji policymakers tested a variety of new chemical insecticides, and this project was closely tied to industrialization. Simply, workers and soldiers needed calories. This interest in insecticides set the Meiji government apart from its early modern predecessor. Through such institutional appendages as the Kaitakushi and agricultural experiment stations situated throughout the country, not to mention a variety of agricultural research organizations, Meiji policymakers directly initiated elaborate national modernization projects and, in the realm of agriculture, established a precedent followed for decades for state-supported insecticide production and deployment. That is, now the modern state, which projected its will through extension agencies and networks and whose representatives rose to power through distinctly Japanese political practices, began altering the natural world. In the modern period, an institutional triad shaped the nature of insecticide production and application: the government, large chemical corporations, and cultivators. Unlike the Tokugawa shogunate, which displayed its support for insect eradication through spells cast at sacred sites, the Meiji government offered resources to a wholly new belief system—science—lending economic support and bringing the technologies and human resources to Japan required for the development of a domestic chemical industry. The case of chrysanthemum-based chemicals is important. In just under two decades, Japan transformed from an importer of "chrysanthemum powder" from England to an exporter of "dried chrysanthemum flowers" to the United States. The same scenario holds true for the production of "parathion" in the 1950s. At first, the chemical giant Sumitomo Chemical imported the highly toxic insecticide from the United States and Germany, but after some prodding by Japanese policymakers concerned with skyrocketing trade deficits after the Allied Occupation, the company began domestic production in earnest by mid-decade.

Not only did nineteenth-century Japan trade ideas, policies, and institutions with Western countries in the name of modernization, it also traded manufactured items such as silk fabric and botanical rarities

such as azaleas, all in the name of global commerce. And similar to the
manner in which Meiji oligarchs winced when they learned that the
democratic writings of Thomas Jefferson (1743–1826) and Jean-Jacques
Rousseau (1712–78) had crept into Japan along with Prussian rumina-
tions on centralized monarchical power, so did American entomologists
when they learned that hungry beetles had hitched rides on azaleas when
Japan exported them to the United States.[47] The saga of the Japanese
beetle occurred as a result of Japan's participation in global commerce,
but the response to the Japanese beetle crisis, as portrayed in our next
case study, reveals a great deal about agricultural policymaking and
cultural attitudes toward insects in Japan and the changing nature of
economic entomology in the United States.

Japanese Invaders

In the early modern period, farmers in western Japan imagined plant
hoppers as the disgruntled spirits of famous medieval warriors and
classical statesmen, even though they traveled to Japan on winds that
originated in southeastern China. Early twentieth-century ecologists in
the United States, operating under a different logic, referred to such foreign insects as "invader species" and took an altogether different
approach to understanding and controlling them. The Japanese beetle
(*Popillia japonica*), known as the "golden coin insect" in western Japan,
invaded the United States in the summer of 1916, when the hungry
chafers established a beachhead at a nursery in Riverton, New Jersey.
When compared to the "helmeted beetles" (*Allomyrina dichotoma*) that
children in Japan collect and raise in small plastic terrariums and whose
shells resemble the ornate armor of medieval samurai warriors, the
Japanese beetle is rather ordinary in everything except for its reflective
golden color and voracious appetite for the same crops that humans tend
to cultivate and eat. Evolution has made it an economic competitor, not
an insect that contributes to human economies, such as silkworms or
even bees. State and federal agencies in the United States, in policy decisions lamented in the pages of Rachel Carson's *Silent Spring*, deployed
insecticides in earnest to kill beetles in mass numbers, chemicals that
later became popular in Japan.

According to economic entomologists, in the first year of its invasion
the beetle inhabited a modest area of about one acre; by 1941, the year
Japanese zeros bombed Pearl Harbor, beetles had made far more impressive gains than Japan's skilled pilots and inhabited some twenty thousand

square miles of soil in the American homeland. East Asian farmers rarely considered the Japanese beetle a serious pest, but once the beetle arrived in New Jersey—its grubs tucked quietly in the bundled roots and soil in a shipment of azaleas—the lack of native predators or diseases meant that it quickly went to work on crops across the country, destroying everything from soybean and clover to apple and peach trees. In the early 1920s, other "Oriental" invader species followed the gains made by the Japanese beetle, including the camphor scale (*Pseudaonidia duplex*) and the Asiatic garden beetle (*Autoserica castanea*).[48] These insects, but mostly the Japanese beetle, represented a scourge on the civilized face of the planet, much as the American propaganda machine famously made out the Japanese people to be once the Pacific War got under way.

By August 1945, even though the United States had subdued, though not eradicated, "Louseous Japanicas" with incendiary bombs and atomic weapons, the Japanese beetle continued to molest crops unimpeded throughout rural America. Rachel Carson featured Japanese beetle eradication campaigns in the Midwest as among the most egregious examples of the dangers of chlorinated hydrocarbons when sprayed indiscriminately over American's pastoral landscapes. Although she did not necessarily identify the campaigns as such, often they exemplified how policy decisions made in institutions, such as in chemical corporations or local and federal government organizations, resonated throughout social networks and ecosystems and, ultimately, harmed human and nonhuman bodies. In 1959, for example, specially equipped airplanes doused about twenty-seven thousand acres in southeastern Michigan with aldrin, a highly toxic and relatively inexpensive insecticide, reportedly to manage the beetle infestation in that area. Despite that fact that some local entomologists questioned the necessity of the program, the aldrin dusting continued apace and, although the beetles survived the bombing, such birds as the American robin did not. Dead songbirds lay strewn around people's lawns. Similarly, between 1954 and 1961, Illinois dusted some 131,000 acres with dieldrin, which, in laboratory tests, proved some fifty times more toxic than the infamous DDT.[49] Here, songbirds and household pets began dying throughout the sprayed areas as well.

What made such campaigns of "annihilation" and "extermination" so tragic is that the Japanese beetle, after about 1954, had, in most instances, ceased to be a serious agricultural pest, as populations had started to stabilize after the initial invasion, largely because of the decision to import new biotechnologies: predatory insects and bacterial "milky" disease from the beetle's native habitat. In retrospect, one can only imagine that, when those

first Japanese beetles made landfall in New Jersey in the earthy roots of
azaleas, they celebrated their arrival in an environment free of at least ten
mortal insect enemies. In Japan, a kind of tachinid fly (*Centeter cinerea*),
through its own reproductive activities, tirelessly kept "golden coin insect"
numbers in check through an ecological equilibrium between the two
species that is centuries old and actually quite gruesome. Indeed, the fly's
unwieldy name in Japanese is Mamekoganeyadoribae, or "the fly that lives
within the Japanese beetle." In their native habitat, among the favorite
haunts of Japanese beetles ranks a variety of knotweed (*Polygonum reynou-
tria*). In this bushy, green world, tachinid flies hunt for unsuspecting (and
usually love-struck) beetles on the leaf tops. So horrified of tachinid flies are
Japanese beetles that if they even catch a glimpse of one they become
alarmed and quickly drop from their leafy cover to the ground rather than
risk confrontation with this ruthless predator. If the fly moves toward the
beetle, sometimes the two engage in a gripping life-or-death struggle.
Tachinid flies have compensated by normally preying on mating beetles,
which usually prove too preoccupied with copulation to notice when the
fly silently stalks them. There is good reason why these small flies scare
Japanese beetles so much. They would you too if you lived in this micro-
scopic world: it is all about scale.

Tachinid flies do not immediately kill and eat the beetles. Instead,
after observing the mating beetles for some time, a female tachinid identifies the female beetle and, in a lightening-fast diagonal run, quickly
maneuvers herself to lay several eggs on the thorax of the female beetle. In
the early 1920s, U.S. researchers from the Bureau of Entomology noticed,
once they arrived in Japan, that in northern parts of the country nearly all
of the Japanese beetles inspected had such eggs around their thorax.
Having attached her eggs to the beetle's thorax—or "provisioned her
eggs"[50]—the female fly's work is basically done; but it serves as a six-day
death sentence for the beetle. The larvae within the eggs develop in about
two days and, rather than hatch externally, the larvae employ rasplike
teeth to bore through the shell of the egg and directly into the thorax of
the beetle. Eggs mistakenly deposited on more armored and, therefore,
better-protected parts of the beetle's exoskeleton often prove unable to
penetrate the body cavity and quickly perish trying. Once in the thoracic
cavity, the larvae molt and then move into the main body cavity, attaching
themselves with a perforated hook to air sacks in order to breathe. The
beetle, being eaten alive from the inside, usually buries itself in the
ground. In the body cavity of the beetle and underground, the larvae then
move back into the thorax, mercifully killing the beetle host in the
process; later, still living inside the beetle, the larvae literally eat the entire

content of the body cavity. Four days after the beetle has died and nine days after the female fly originally attached her eggs, the larvae metamorphose into a pupa and survive in the buried cavity until they emerge in the early morning hours some ten months later. Once mature, the female flies then search for another love-struck female beetle on whom to lay their eggs and procreate. The engineers at chemical giant American Cyanamid could never have even dreamt up such an effective insect-killing machine, particularly one with so little collateral damage. Because of the tachinid fly and other predatory insects, Japanese beetles never posed much of a threat to Japanese farmers, unless, of course, these farmers unwittingly used chemicals that killed tachinids, which they often did.

Starting in 1921, the team from the Bureau of Entomology (part of the U.S. Department of Agriculture) paid over two hundred Japanese children to collect parasitized specimens of the Japanese beetle to be shipped to the United States and released at ground zero in Riverton, New Jersey. The Japanese kids must have had a blast making money in their age-old hobby of netting insects. As far back as the early eleventh century, Japanese courtiers wrote nostalgically of the ringing songs of the bell cricket (*Homoeogryllus japonicus*), which they described poetically and, in typical Japanese fashion, onomatopoeically. Courtiers sometimes collected these emotionally evocative insects and then set them free in their gardens. Tachibana Narisue, in his *Kokon Chomonju* (Notable tales old and new) described children meeting in 1095 in the fields of Saga near Kyoto to catch insects. Everybody from the head priest downward gathered horses from official pavilions and departed the capital with stylized bamboo cages with dangling decorative cords. The party dismounted at Toyomachi and proceeded on foot. They caught insects until evening and then returned to the capital, where they fed the crickets and other creeping creatures leaves from bush clover and a perennial plant with yellow flowers (*Patrinia scabiosaefolia*). Once back in the palace, the courtiers raised their saké cups and composed poetry regarding the occasion.[51] The fictional Prince Genji had autumn insects released into his garden in order to create a lonely mood that evoked, as Heian courtiers were want to do, a Buddhist sense of impermanence and, as we have seen, transcendence.[52]

Later, in the eighteenth and early nineteenth centuries, the admirers of insect songs learned how to cultivate crickets in how-to books. Raising the eggs of the pine cricket (*Xenogryllus marmorata*) proved relatively simple and something that any enthusiast could do.[53] The ability to cultivate insects led to the business of insect vendors (*mushi uri*) in some towns and cities. In the nineteenth century as well, Kitagawa Morisada described the practice of selling insects as one of the "modern customs" of Tokugawa Japan. On city streets, decorative bamboo cages dangling from colorful insect-vendor kiosks contained singing bell crickets (*Homoeogryllus japonicus*), giant katydids (*Mecopoda elongata*), pine crickets (*Xenogryllus marmorata*), buprestid beetles (*Chrysochroa fulgidissima*), and many others.[54]

So, historically speaking, Japanese kids and their parents knew something about collecting and keeping bugs, because it was part of Japan's cultural heritage. U.S. entomologists tapped into this historical expertise to collect and deploy their biotechnologies. By 1924, after releasing beetles with eggs around their thoraxes, entomologists spotted parasitized Japanese beetles within a twelve-mile radius of Riverton.[55] The policy decision was a success: the fate of the Japanese beetle in the United States was sealed, but chemical companies and their political allies still pushed hard for the use of chemical insecticides, both in the United States and abroad.

The Age of Chemical Insecticides

Chlorinated hydrocarbons and organophosphates caught on in Japan after the Pacific War. Whale oil was an insecticidal technology gained from boiling the blubber of whales; deploying tachinid flies, by contrast, was entirely an issue of overcoming island biogeographies and transporting the predatory insects to the United States. Postwar insecticides proved altogether different in the manner that they interacted with insect bodies and the environment, and these chemicals provide our final case study.

The utterly lethal organophosphorus ester insecticide "parathion" ranked among the most deadly poisons in the world and among the favorites of Japan's postwar farmers, pesticide companies, and, somewhat surprisingly, people who sought to commit suicide or even homicide.[56] As Linda Nash has shown, it was a favorite among the fruit growers of California as well. As early as 1949, California farmers applied parathion to their fields and orchards; that same year, in Marysville, California, twenty-five migrant workers became seriously ill after entering an orchard prayed previously with parathion. Nash has stressed nature's unanticipated agency when it comes to the toxicity and human-health threat represented by such chemicals. Nash writes, "A study of parathion decay conducted in the 1970s revealed that pesticide residues in the same fields could vary as much as 90-fold, depending upon the time of year the chemical was applied." In other words, "Once introduced into the environment, OP (organophosphate) chemicals were subject to the uncontrolled agency of nature."[57] Of course, this is precisely the nature of the unanticipated, unforeseen "eco-system" accidents described by Perrow at the outset of this article.

In Japan, parathion injured people and environments in a similar fashion, but it also did so according to unanticipated, social system (as opposed to just eco-system) accidents. That a government warning of the dangers of parathion's extreme toxicity served to alert those who wanted to commit suicide of its effectiveness is a wonderful—if incredibly grim— example of the unanticipated manner in which policy decisions and information crosscut different social networks to say different things and have different consequences to different people. Ironically, but not surprisingly, the numerous suicides resulting from consuming parathion and its relative biocide paraquat are systematically related to government and corporate efforts to stem accidental exposure to the insecticide through the dissemination of information regarding its toxic qualities.

The German chemist Gerhard Schrader developed the first organophosphate chemicals at the Farbenfabriken Bayer AG facilities in 1937 and the Nazis merrily continued their development as a chemical weapon. Although several generations removed, parathion is related to sarin gas, which the Japanese cult Aum Shinrikyo, led by its spiritual leader Asahara Shoko, used to murder twelve and injure thousands of Tokyo subway riders in March 1995. Chemists developed parathion in 1944 and it began replacing DDT in the 1950s, mainly because of its suitability as an insecticide: it persisted well in the environment and did not break down in sunlight or water.[58] Obviously, these same resilient qualities made it a dangerous environmental polluter—it haunts environments for ages, not to mention that it morphs into even deadlier forms under nature's unantici- pated auspices.

When Japanese farmers began spraying parathion on their rice crops in the 1950s, they noticed quick results and yields soared. One doctor overoptimistically boasted that, as a result of parathion, Japan's perennial postwar food shortage had been "solved." But better yields came at a high cost: in a period of six years, between 1953 and 1958, physicians reported nearly ten thousand instances of parathion poisoning and three thousand of those proved fatal.[59] Basically, parathion, as with all organophosphates, is a cholinesterase inhibiter and so, in larger doses, it can kill and, in smaller doses, it can injure reproduction; the symptoms include muscle twitching (fasciculation), breathing difficulties, profuse sweating, and urinary and fecal problems.[60] It should not be surprising, then, that early on some Japanese researchers suspected parathion as being responsible for fetal deaths and other difficulties. In the 1950s, the Japanese government distributed some fifty thousand grams of moderately successful "oxime" therapy around the country to treat potential cases of parathion poisoning. With one treatment requiring between one and two grams per patient, the Japanese government, we can assume, anticipated tens of thousands of cases of accidental poisoning.[61]

Originally, farmers used parathion to kill rice-eating bugs, such as Asiatic rice borers (Chilo suppressalis), stinkbugs (Pentatomidae), and plant hoppers, but policymakers also targeted fruit and vegetables eaters, such as aphides and leaf folders. The Japanese imported parathion from Bayer and American Cyanamid in the form of an emulsion (a liquid that is a mixture of one or more liquids) in 1951. Quickly, the Ministry of Agriculture and Forestry hailed the effectiveness of the chemical against the Asiatic rice borer and appropriated 40 million yen for experiments in mass extermination. But because parathion is extremely poisonous, two high-profile incidents alerted people to its dangers: a girl from Shizuoka prefecture and an agricultural reform advocate from Hyogo prefecture died from parathion poisoning.[62] In response, lawmakers passed ordinances to alert people to parathion's toxicity.

Originally, the government passed the Agricultural Chemical Control Law (Noyaku torishimari no hosei) in 1948 less to prohibit the circulation of illegal, highly toxic, or poor-quality chemicals than simply to increase production and improve their quality. As Gerald Markowitz and David Rosner document in the United States, big chemical companies, not victims of chemical poisons, had the undivided attention of policymakers and the same was true in Japan.[63] But the government voiced good intentions and its statement is worth quoting, because of the similarities to the case of the United States. According to the Japanese government: "This law establishes a registry system for agricultural chemicals and, more than act to control their sale and use, to promote safety it normalizes the quality of agricultural chemicals and ensures proper use of them. It also stabilizes the production of agricultural chemicals and contributes to the protection of the health of the citizenry, together with contributing to the preservation of the living environment of the citizenry."[64] Ultimately, the law would be revised on three occasions (1951, 1962, and 1963); and it was not until October 1972 that it was given any real teeth by what is called the "Pollution Diet." Five years after the original law, the Welfare and Agriculture and Forestry ministries started enacting tougher "control laws" to educate people about the dangers of agricultural products, particularly parathion and methyl parathion. In August 1955 the government listed parathion as a "special poison" (tokutei dokubutsu), one year after Sumitomo Chemical began its domestic manufacture.[65]

Unabashedly, Sumitomo's corporate histories published as late as the 1980s gush that the development of parathion provided a "valuable service" to "our country." According to these histories, Sumitomo discovered the economic promise of parathion in July 1950 after the company president, Doi Masaharu, visited the headquarters of American Cyanamid. In September of the next year, American Cyanamid sought to establish international economic ties to Japan and tapped Sumitomo to peddle the chemical in East Asia more broadly. Initially, the strategy was that American Cyanamid would offer Sumitomo parathion to sell in Asia and, over time, nurture a robust market for the insecticide. Then, once market share had been created, Sumitomo would be taught how to manufacture the chemical itself. In June 1951, at about the same time that American Cyanamid tried to expand the parathion market in East Asia, Bayer began marketing "Folidol"—their proprietary name for parathion— in Japan as well. Subsequent tests in agricultural experiment stations proved that the chemical killed Asiatic rice borers in rice paddies, dry-land crops, and fruit orchards. Not surprisingly, policymakers quickly approved Folidol for use in Japan. Its toxic effectiveness was a far cry from the whale-oil insecticides of the Kyoho famine, but so was the effectiveness of the institutional systems through which it disseminated from chemical corporations to agricultural lands to human bodies.

Meanwhile, the Sumitomo relationship with American Cyanamid continued to solidify. In March 1952, Sumitomo became American Cyanamid's "Japan delegate" for the marketing and manufacture of parathion; later, in September of that same year, the two companies jointly decided that Sumitomo would construct factories in Japan to manufacture parathion but that, until that time, Sumitomo would import and sell the American product. By November 1953, Sumitomo was importing and selling American Cyanamid's product. Importantly, there was a slight difference between the parathion produced by American Cyanamid and Bayer: the former manufactured ethyl parathion, while the latter produced methyl parathion. Comparatively speaking, ethyl parathion is more toxic, though both, if handled improperly (or even properly), can prove deadly.[66] To Sumitomo, the Bayer product appeared more appropriate to Japan's small farms and so the company sought a licensing agreement with Bayer; but immediate postwar economic conditions in Japan prompted the government to try to limit the number of imports and begin more domestic production and this extended to the chemical industry as well. With the government urging Sumitomo to begin the immediate domestic production of parathion, the Japanese company acquired licenses to manufacture

American Cyanamid's product in May 1953 and Bayer's product a bit later, in October 1953.

Production began at Sumitomo's Tsurusaki plant. The site proved optimal for two reasons: the company already stored the raw material paranitrochloro benzene (PNCB) at the site, and facilities at the site that had once produced monochloro benzene (but had been idle since 1951) could be put back to use for the company. By March 1954, at the Tsurusaki plant, Sumitomo began the monthly production of some thirty tons of ethyl parathion. To boost production still, Sumitomo's Okayama Plant, which produced monochloro benzene, an ingredient in ethyl parathion, was fully automated for remote operation. By March 1955, Sumitomo had begun the production of Bayer's methyl parathion at the Tsurusaki site was well. That year, Sumitomo manufactured some fifty tons of ethyl and methyl parathion at the Tsurusaki plant.

In April 1955, Sumitomo manufactured enough parathion to halt importing the chemical from the United States and, in time, it supplied all Japanese domestic consumption of the pesticide. Manufacture of the insecticide expanded at a staggering pace: in 1955, the Tsurusaki plant boasted a monthly production of 630 tons; by 1960 that number had increased to 1,000 tons. Starting in September 1957, Sumitomo marketed parathion throughout Japan under the Bayer name Folidol. Simultaneously, Sumitomo established the Parathion Research Group (Parachion Kenkyukai) in 1954 and, presumably in response to the highly toxic nature of the insecticide, the Parathion Poisoning Remedy Research Group (Parachion Chudoku Chiryoho Kenkyukai) in 1955.[67] Parathion became nothing less than a ubiquitous part of Japan's chemical industry and agrarian landscapes, from dry-land crops and orchards to terraced paddies. But once in the fields, eco-system accidents and social system accidents began to occur in a manner that few advocates or critics of the chemical could have anticipated.

To be sure, hundreds of people died as a result of accidental poisonings. But in a ghoulish twist, in Japan policy decisions to warn people of accidental poisoning by parathion proved to be part of the public-health threat posed by the insecticide. In 1956, one year after policymakers designated parathion as a "special toxin," accidental death rates plummeted from eighty-six people to twenty-nine. That same year, however, the use of parathion for suicides or as a murder weapon nearly doubled. Obviously, the designation "special toxin" possessed two voices that emerged when it crosscut different social networks: it served to warn some and advertise to others.

The use of parathion and related agricultural chemicals for suicide is striking. Japan remains a country that stresses social conformity that has, according to some specialists, contributed to its dubious distinction of having one of the highest suicide rates in the industrialized world. In the 1950s, the ingestion of large doses of parathion was one method of choice for those hoping to end their lives. By the 1980s, however, the herbicide known as paraquat had become the poison of choice. Chemists developed paraquat in 1882, but its propensity to kill pests was not discovered until 1959. This bipyridyl herbicide ranks among the most deadly pulmonary poisons known and so has attracted an enormous amount of scientific attention.[68] Basically, paraquat releases oxygen-fee radicals that painfully destroy lung and kidney tissue. In Japan, the number of suicidal, homicidal, and accidental deaths from paraquat increased steadily in the mid-1980s: from 594 in 1984 to 1,021 in 1985. Of the 1,021 deaths reported in 1985, over 96 percent of those proved suicidal. What made young people contemplating suicide aware of its lethal properties was a series of indiscriminate, and highly sensationalized, soft-drink poisonings that left seventeen dead in 1985; another reason was that, in the 1980s, paraquat was readily available in Japanese garden shops and unwittingly advertised as a "special toxin" by the Japanese government. Today, the Japanese government has severely restricted the chemical to only those people with proper documentation and laced the herbicide with vivid colors and rancid odors to make it less palatable to those who might drink it.[69]

Conclusion

As early as March 1966, Japan's Diet began taking steps against certain toxic insecticides, such as phenyl-mercury; even earlier, the Ministry of Agriculture and Forestry, in both May 1965 and May 1966, had directed that nonmercuric pesticides replace mercuric ones.[70] By December 1969, the government suspended the production of parathion and TEPP; by the summer of that same year, even the sale of ethyl and methyl parathion had been prohibited. Sumitomo histories explain that the suspension of parathion production was caused by two factors: pesky insects such as the Asiatic rice borer had developed evolutionary resistances to the chemical, and it killed or poisoned too many people. But between 1954 and 1969, for a period of sixteen years, 6,648 tons of ethyl parathion and 3,960 tons of methyl parathion—a total of 10,608 tons sprayed throughout Japan—had been manufactured and sold in Japan.[71]

Soon thereafter, in May 1971, the government prohibited the sale of DDT, while sales of BHC, endrin, dieldrin, and aldrin were restricted. One month later, the government prohibited the use of parathion, methyl parathion, and TEPP.[72] In 1972, the government passed a series of laws prohibiting or seriously restricting many highly toxic agricultural chemicals.

What these six case studies tell us about the interrelationships among government and corporate policy decisions, social networks, cultural sensibilities, toxic chemicals, and Japan's ecosystems is that policy history needs to be placed in broader contexts. When it comes to chlorinated hydrocarbons or organophosphates, derelict policy decisions are not just derelict policy decisions; they are decisions that resonate throughout the natural and unnatural systems in which human populations remain deeply imbedded. Policy decisions, when amplified through hybridized systems, cause evolution in the form of hereditary resistances among resilient insect populations, unanticipated ecosystem accidents in highly engineered agricultural landscapes, epidemic disease as a result of anthropogenic biogeographic proximity (i.e., proximity among pigs, humans, and mosquitoes), and health problems among human consumers who, when at the dinner table, interface directly with all these "trophic" (food-chain) layers.

That is, not all evolution is a result of chance. The policy decisions humans conjure—whether economically driven to cull certain silkworms or designed to situate piggeries near cities and their cemeteries for access to garbage, or religiously driven to combat pesky insects through spells, or scientifically driven to manufacture more lethal biocides—are broadcast through natural systems and directly affect human and nonhuman health.

Montana State University,
Bozeman

Notes

1 This subfield of environmental history is often called "envirotech." As the name suggests, it bridges scholarship in the history of technology and environmental history. See Timothy LeCain, "What Is Envirotech? Some Emergent Properties of a New Historical Subfield," *The Envirotech Newsletter* 5 (2005): 1, 4–5.

2. The intriguing argument that human enterprises, such as industry, science, and technology, have so transformed nature that the planet no longer exists in its previously recognizable form, whatever that might have been for people, is articulated nicely in Bill McKibben, *The End of Nature* (New York, 1997).

3. See chapter one of my *The Lost Wolves of Japan*, foreword by William Cronon (Seattle, 2005). In many respects, the morphological development of the Japanese wolf, *C.l. hodophilax*, and hence its taxonomic designation, was the product of anthropogenic environmental forces in Japan's early modern and modern histories.

4. Edmund Russell, "Evolutionary History: Prospectus for a New Field," *Environmental History* 8 (April 2003): 205-6.

5. On the "big chicken" industry in the United States, see Steve Striffler, *Chicken: The Dangerous Transformation of America's Favorite Food* (New Haven, 2005).

6. Michael Pollan has discussed the theme of "co-evolution" in relationship to certain desirable plants in *The Botany of Desire: A Plant's-Eye View of the World* (New York, 2002).

7. Edmund Russell, "Introduction: The Garden in the Machine: Toward an Evolutionary History of Technology," in *Industrializing Organisms: Introducing Evolutionary History*, ed. Susan R. Schrepfer and Philip Scranton, Hagley Perspectives on Business and Culture, vol. 5 (New York, 2004), 1, 4, 8, 11, 13.

8. Pete Daniel, *Toxic Drift: Pesticides and Health in the Post-World War II South* (Baton Rouge, 2005).

9. Joshua Blu Buhs, *The Fire Ant Wars: Nature, Science, and Public Policy in Twentieth-Century America* (Chicago, 2004).

10. Jonathan Weiner explores some insect resistances in *The Beak of the Finch* (New York, 1994), 253-55.

11. Deborah Kay Fitzgerald, *Every Farm a Factory: The Industrial Ideal in American Agriculture* (New Haven, 2003).

12. For an excellent treatment of forms of biomagnification, see Sandra Steingraber, *Having Faith: An Ecologist's Journey to Motherhood* (Cambridge, 2001).

13. Charles Perrow, *Normal Accidents: Living with High-Risk Technologies* (New York, 1984; repr., Princeton, 1999), 14, 233, 295, 296.

14. On social networks, see John F. Padgett and Christopher K. Ansell, "Robust Action and the Rise of the Medici, 1400-1434," *American Journal of Sociology* 98, no. 6 (May 1993): 1259-65. As for ecosystems, the British plant ecologist Arthur Tansley coined the term "ecosystem" in 1935. He wrote that "the whole *system* (in the sense of physics) including not only the organism-complex, but also the whole complex of physical factors forming what we call the environment of the biome—the habitat factors in the widest sense." See Robert P. McIntosh, *The Background of Ecology: Concepts and Theory* (Cambridge, 1985), 193.

15. Marian R. Goldsmith, Toru Shimada, and Hiroaki Abe, "The Genetics and Genomics of the Silkworm, Bombyx mori," *Annual Review of Entomology* 50 (January 2005): 71-100.

16. A standard treatment of Heian Japanese aesthetics and cultural sensibilities is Ivan Morris, *The World of the Shining Prince: Court Life in Ancient Japan* (New York, 1964).

17. Goldsmith, Shimada, and Abe, "The Genetics and Genomics of the Silkworm," 71-100.

18. Kasai Masaaki, *Mushi to Nihon bunka* (Insects and Japanese culture) (Tokyo, 1997), 72-73.

19. *Kojiki* (Record of Ancient Matters), translated with an introduction and notes by Donald L. Philippi (Tokyo, 1968), 87.

20. Ibid., 313.

21. Brett L. Walker, "Commercial Growth and Environmental Change in Early Modern Japan: Hachinohe's Wild Boar Famine of 1749," *Journal of Asian Studies* 60, no. 2 (Spring 2001): 329-51.

22. Simon Partner, *Toshié: A Story of Village Life in Twentieth-Century Japan* (Berkeley and Los Angeles, 2004), 17-20.

23. An excellent treatment of early modern Japanese rural lending institutions is Ronald P. Toby, "Both a Borrower and a Lender Be: From Village Moneylender to Rural Banker in the Tempō Era," *Monumenta Nipponica* 46, no. 4 (Winter 1991): 483-512. In

the context of Japan's "household system," it fell on the shoulders of peasant women such as Matsuo Taseko to care for silkworms and thereby elevate the wealth of their husbands' households. See Anne Walthall, *The Weak Body of a Useless Woman: Matsuo Taseko and the Meiji Restoration* (Chicago, 1998).

24. For example, Lady Nijo lamented the death of her lover, the emperor, with a poem that referred to the seasonal (and hence representative of transient) calls of insects and deer. See *The Confessions of Lady Nijo*, trans. Karen Brazell (Stanford, 1973).

25. David B. Lurie, "Orientomology: The Insect Literature of Lafcadio Hearn (1850-1904)," in *JAPANimals: History and Culture in Japan's Animal Life*, ed. Gregory M. Pflugfelder and Brett L. Walker (Ann Arbor, 2005), 245-62.

26. Lafcadio Hearn, *Kwaidan: Stories and Studies of Strange Things* (Boston, 1904; repr., Rutland, Vt., 1971), 184, 207-12.

27. In 1900, Japanese built 1,396 slaughterhouses throughout their country. At these slaughterhouses, between 1893 and 1902, employees dispatched over 1.7 million cattle to fuel the workers and soldiers of modern Japan. Pigs were an important industrialized organism as well. See The Department of Agriculture and Commerce, ed. *Japan in the Beginning of the 20th Century* (Tokyo, 1904), 184-200.

28. "The Livestock Industry of Japan," Report Number 30, General Headquarters, Supreme Commander for the Allied Powers, Natural Resources Section, APO 500, 18 April 1944.

29. John W. Dower, *Embracing Defeat: Japan in the Wake of World War II* (New York, 1999), 133.

30. Daniel Barenblatt, *A Plague upon Humanity: The Hidden History of Japan's Biological Warfare Program* (New York, 2004), 9-10.

31. "Japanese Use the Chinese as 'Guinea Pigs' to Test Germ Warfare," *Rocky Mountain Medical Journal* 39, no. 8 (August 1942): 571-72; *Materials on the Trial of Former Servicemen of the Japanese Army Charged with Manufacturing and Employing Bacteriological Weapons* (Moscow, 1950); John W. Powell, "A Hidden Chapter in History," *The Bulletin of the Atomic Scientists* 37, no. 8 (October 1981): 49-50.

32. Edmund P. Russell, "'Speaking of Annihilation': Mobilization for War Against Human and Insect Enemies, 1914-1945," *Journal of American History* 82, no. 4 (March 1996): 1505-6, 1508, 1511, 1522-27. On the dehumanization of the enemy, both in the United States and Japan, see John W. Dower, *War Without Mercy: Race and Power in the Pacific War* (New York, 1986).

33. Buddhist beliefs provide one reason why Japanese cultivators believed that talismans from shrines such as Mt. Zozu's Konpira, on Shikoku Island, prevented serious insect damage. See Sarah Thal, *Rearranging the Landscape of the Gods: The Politics of a Pilgrimage Site in Japan, 1573-1912* (Chicago, 2005), 106-7.

34. J. H. Mun, Y. H. Song, K. L. Heong, and G. K. Roderick, "Genetic Variation among Asian Populations of Rice Planthoppers, *Nilaparvata lugens* and *Sogatella furcifera* (Hemiptera: Delphacidae): Mitochondrial DNA Sequences," *Bulletin of Entomological Research* 89 (1999): 245-53.

35. In what is called the *kokudaka* system, the Tokugawa regime measured the wealth of feudal domains and their retainers according to an amount called *koku*, wherein one *koku* equaled 5.1 bushels of rice. The philosophy behind this amount was that one *koku* of rice could feed a human for one year.

36. *The Ten Foot Square Hut and Tales of the Heike*, trans. A. L. Sadler (Sydney, 1928), 123-24.

37. Robert Borgen, *Suguwara no Michizane and the Early Heian Court* (Honolulu, 1986), 278-325.

38. For more on whaling in Japan, see Arne Kalland and Brian Moeran, *Japanese Whaling: End of an Era?* (London, 1992). See also Arne Kalland, *Fishing Villages in Tokugawa Japan* (Honolulu, 1995).

39. Kikuchi Isao, *Kinsei no kikin* (Early modern Japan's famines) (Tokyo, 1997), 82-89.

40. Conrad Totman, *Early Modern Japan* (Berkeley and Los Angeles, 1993), 236–38.

41. Once again, these two terms refer to Japanese imperial reign names. The Tenmei period lasted from 1781 to 1788; the Tenpo period lasted from 1830 to 1843.

42. The need to get more productivity out of rural lands with fewer laborers also led to the development of nitrogenous fertilizers. See Barbara Molony, *Technology and Investment: The Prewar Japanese Chemical Industry* (Cambridge, Mass., 1990), 17–266. For more recent data on fertilizer use, see David Vogel, "Consumer Protection and Protectionism in Japan," *Journal of Japanese Studies* 18, no. 1 (Winter 1992): 131–32.

43. The Meiji Japanese adoption and adaptation of Euro-American science is covered in James R. Bartholomew, *The Formation of Science in Japan* (New Haven, 1989).

44. On the role of foreign experts in refashioning Hokkaido and agricultural practices there, see Hokkaido Prefectural Government, ed. *Foreign Pioneers: A Short History of the Contribution of Foreigners to the Development of Hokkaido* (Sapporo, 1968). See also Fumiko Fujita, *American Pioneers and the Japanese Frontier: American Experts in Nineteenth-Century Japan* (Westport, Conn., 1994); John M. Maki, *William Smith Clark: A Yankee in Hokkaido* (Sapporo, 1996).

45. James Whorton, *Before Silent Spring: Pesticides and Public Health in Pre-DDT America* (Princeton, 1974), 8–9, 12, 15–16, 20, 22, 64–65.

46. Matsunaka Shoichi, *Nihon ni okeru noyaku no rekishi* (Japan's agricultural chemical history) (Tokyo, 2002), 9–11. For more specific information on plant disease, insects, and insecticides from the Meiji period through the 1950s, see Tennensha Jiten Henshubu, ed. *Byochu noyaku jiten* (Dictionary of agricultural chemicals for disease and insects) (Tokyo, 1955).

47. Historian Irokawa Daikichi famously discovered a draft, nineteenth-century constitution, written by commoners, tucked in the attic of a rural farmhouse. The writings of Jefferson and Rousseau inspired much of the unofficial document. See Daikichi Irokawa, *The Culture of the Meiji Period*, trans. Marius Jansen (Princeton, 1988). Nonetheless, Ito Hirobumi and his advisers, when drafting the official Meiji Constitution of 1889, relied mostly on Prussian monarchical theories. See Carol Gluck, *Japan's Modern Myths: Ideology in the Late Meiji Period* (Princeton, 1985).

48. Charles S. Elton, *The Ecology of Invasions by Animals and Plants* (London, 1958; repr., Chicago, 2000), 52–54.

49. Aldrin and dieldrin are closely related chemicals that fall under the cyclodiene classification of chlorinated hydrocarbons. Once sprayed in the environment, both chemicals bioconcentrate and biomagnify in a manner that kills or inhibits the reproductive success of many nonhuman species, especially in avian species.

50. David Quammen, *Monster of God: The Man-eating Predator in the Jungles of History and the Mind* (New York, 2003), 426–27.

51. Tachibana Narisue, *Kokon chomonju* (Notable tales old and new), vol. 2, in *Shincho Nihon koten shusei* (Shincho collection of classical Japanese literature), vol. 76, ed. Nishio Koichi and Kobayashi Yasuharu (Tokyo, 1986), 372. For a description of this collection, see Yoshiko K. Dykstra, "Notable Tales Old and New: Tachibana Narisue's *Kokon Chomonju*," *Monumenta Nipponica* 47, no. 4 (Winter 1992): 469–93.

52. Murasaki Shikibu, *The Tale of Genji*, trans. and with intro. by Edward G. Seidensticker (New York, 1997), 671.

53. *Churyo manroku*, cited in Kasai, *Mushi to Nihon bunka*, 132–33.

54. Kitagawa Morisada, *Ruiju kinsei fuzokushi* (Record of various modern customs), ed. Muromatsu Iwao (Tokyo, 1928), 167.

55. Curtis P. Clausen, J. L. King, and Cho Teranishi, "The Parasites of *Popillia Japonica* in Japan and Chosen (Korea), and Their Introduction into the United States," *United States Department of Agriculture Department Bulletin* 1429 (January 1927): 1–55.

56. See, for example, Watanabe Yuji, *Kurashi ni hisomu kagaku dokubutsu jiten* (A Dictionary of chemical poisons that lurk in our daily lives) (Tokyo, 2002), 74; Nakaminami Gen, *Noyaku genron* (The principles of agricultural chemicals) (Tokyo, 2001), 23–25; Miura

Yoshiaki, *Kagaku osen to ningen no rekishi* (Chemical contamination and human history) (Tokyo, 1999), 73-74; Yasuhara Akio, *Shinobi yoru kagaku busshitsu osen: Chikyu tanjo, seitaikei, gendai bunmei ni okeru kagaku busshitsu osen no keifu* (Exposing chemical contamination: The birth of earth, ecological structure, and the genealogy of chemical contamination in the context of modern civilizatation) (Tokyo, 1999), 143-45; Ando Mitsuru, *Yokuwakaru noyaku osen: Jintai to kankyo o mushibamu gosei kagaku busshitsu* (Agricultural chemical contamination: The synthetic chemical compounds that ruin human bodies and the environment) (Tokyo, 1990), 21-25.

57. Linda Nash, "The Fruits of Ill-Health: Pesticides and Workers' Bodies in Post-World War II California," *Osiris* 19 (2004): 205, 208. See also Linda Nash, "Finishing Nature: Harmonizing Bodies and Environments in Late-Nineteenth-Century California," *Environmental History* 8 (January 2003): 25-52.

58. Curtis D. Klaassen, ed. *Casarett & Doull's Toxicology: The Basic Science of Poisons*, 5th ed. (New York, 1996), 655.

59. Tatsuji Namba, "Oxime Therapy for Poisoning by Alkylphosphate-Insecticides," *Proceedings of the 13th Annual International Congress on Occupational Health, July 25-29, 1960* (1961): 757.

60. Takashi Tanimura, "Embryotoxicity of Acute Exposure to Methyl Parathion in Rats and Mice," *Archives of Environmental Health* 15 (November 1967): 609-13.

61. Namba, "Oxime Therapy for Poisoning by Alkylphosphate-Insecticides," 757-58.

62. Uemura Shinsaku, Kawamura Hiroshi, Tsuji Machiko, Tomita Shigeyuki, and Maeda Shizuo, *Noyaku dokusei no jiten* (Dictionary of toxic agricultural chemicals) (Tokyo, 2002), 146-47.

63. Gerald Markowitz and David Rosner, *Deceit and Denial: The Deadly Politics of Industrial Pollution* (Berkeley and Los Angeles, 2002).

64. Kankyo Horei Kenkyukai, ed. *Kankyo kogai nenkan* (Yearbook of environmental public damage) (Tokyo, 1973), 137.

65. Shimokawa Koshi, ed. *Kankyoshi nenpyo: Showa-Heisei hen* (Environmental history chronology: Showa and Heisei periods), vol. 2 (Tokyo, 2004), 193.

66. For some examples of the deadly consequences of parathion use, see Daniel, *Toxic Drift*, 108-24.

67. Sumitomo Kagaku Kogyo Kabushikigaisha, ed. *Sumitomo Kagaku Kogyo Kabushikigaisha shi* (A history of Sumitomo Chemical) (Osaka, 1981), 305-9.

68. Klaassen, ed., *Casarett & Doull's Toxicology*, 673.

69. Yoshimoto Takahashi, Hideto Hirasawa, and Keiko Koyama, "Restriction of Suicide Methods: A Japanese Perspective," *Archives of Suicide Research* 4 (1998): 103-4.

70. The fixation with mercury was in part due to the outbreak of "Minamata disease," or methyl-mercury poisoning, in southern Japan. See Norie Huddle and Michael Reich with Nahum Stiskin, *Island of Dreams: Environmental Crisis in Japan*, foreword by Dr. Paul R. Ehrlich and afterword by Ralph Nader (New York, 1975), 102-32; Frank K. Upham, *Law and Social Change in Postwar Japan* (Cambridge, Mass., 1989), 28-77; Jun Ui, *Industrial Pollution in Japan* (Tokyo, 1992), 103-32; and Timothy S. George, *Minamata: Pollution and the Struggle for Democracy in Postwar Japan* (Cambridge, Mass., 2001). On the pathology of "Minamata disease," see Masazumi Harada with Aileen M. Smith, "Minamata Disease: A Medical Report," in W. Eugene Smith and Aileen M. Smith, *Minamata* (New York, 1975), 180-92; Tadao Tsubaki and Katsuro Irukayama, ed. *Minamata Disease: Methylmercury Poisoning in Minamata and Niigata, Japan* (Tokyo and Amsterdam, 1977); Tadao Takeuchi and Komyo Eto, *The Pathology of Minamata Disease: A Tragic Story of Water Pollution* (Fukuoka, 1999).

71. Sumitomo Kagaku Kogyo Kabushikigaisha, ed. *Sumitomo Kagaku Kogyo Kabushikigaisha shi*, 543-44.

72. Shimokawa, ed. *Kankyoshi nenpyo: Showa-Heisei hen*, 283.